Praise for *Progr*

"Good science is not lacking to use lifestyle as medicine, and add years to lives and life to years; what holds us back is lack of good sense about applying the science available to us. Just such sense is on abundant display here, and I applaud Gregg Roberts for making it accessible to all."
— *Dr. David L. Katz, MD, MPH, FACPM, FACP Founding Director of Yale University's Prevention Research Center at Griffin Hospital/President of the American College of Lifestyle Medicine*

"I'm a family doctor and a mother. While I try to practice what I preach to my patients, I realize I'm still not doing enough to help myself and my family feel better and live healthier. Finally, a book that breaks down the secret to better living in easy steps and eating cleaner!"
— *Dr. Lisa Melnychuk, South Salem, NY*

"I believe we have the power to stop managing symptoms and start treating the root cause of sickness. In his book, Gregg gives you a series of simple steps that underscore this belief, backed by science, that will guide you on your journey toward a healthier life. Transforming your health is in your control."
— *Dr. Mark Hyman, Medical Director at Cleveland Clinic's Center for Functional Medicine, the Founder of The UltraWellness Center, and a ten-time #1 New York Times Bestselling author*

"In *PROGRESS OVER PERFECTION*, Gregg Roberts has done all the research for you and streamlined how to better your lifestyle and health. Take a journey with him and you will feel better and live longer!"
— *Shannon McGinn, Producer, "Profiles Television" & "The Amazing Race"*

"So often our resolve to eat and feel better comes unraveled as each imperfect choice slowly erodes our will. We find ourselves slipping back to our poor, easy, non-nutritious habits. In *Progress Over Perfection*, Gregg Roberts lays out an easy to follow guide to better health. The title says it all, make a good choice right now, that's Progress. Perfection exists in the imagination of what your life and health can be, by slowly, routinely building your life's new routine of healthy eating."

—*Al Cafaro former Chairman and CEO of A&M Records*

"Running a business is hard, taxing stuff. This books makes it easy to make small changes with big impact in how we live our lives. I've seen meaningful results in my life."

—*Seth Besmertnik CEO, Conductor*

"Being deeply involved in the fitness industry, it is clear to me just how unaware and misinformed so many people are regarding nutrition and wellness. *Progress Over Perfection* is inspirational and written in an easily digestible way that includes lessons I will continue to share with my own sons. The healthcare system in the US is a mess, but our own health and wellbeing does not need to be! Kudos to Mr. Roberts for his clearly stated strategies."

—*Steve Schnall, Co-Chairman Fit Athletic Holdings &*
CEO/Chairman Quontic Bank

"As a father of five young children, the health and wellness of my family is everything to me. Between my parenting responsibilities and travel schedule, I don't always get the time to read as much as I would like, so I appreciate the simple, yet evidence based presentation of *Progress Over Perfection*. It's an easy, light read packed with invaluable tools and resources to live a healthier life."

—*Greg Young Founder & Chairman, BeFoundation*

"I have always worked out at the gym and figured that was enough to keep me healthy. What *Progress Over Perfection* taught me was that there is more to being healthy than just hitting the gym and watching my calories. This book is full of simple tools to help me attain great results without adhering to a rigid diet or lifestyle regimen."

—Matt Shendell Founder Paige Hospitality Group

"I've had some recent health challenges due to a hectic schedule and not necessarily paying as much attention to my own wellness. Gregg's straightforward book on a very important topic is sure to light a spark within me to make some of those small, yet necessary changes to my lifestyle so I can begin taking better control of my own health. *Progress Over Perfection* contains valuable wisdom for those of us looking to be proactive instead of reactive when it comes to our health and wellbeing."

—Dr. Clive Calver, Author, Pastor,
and Former President of World Relief

"Gregg's book is perfect for anyone who wants to optimize their health long term and avoid chronic disease. He synthesizes the best information and research available into simple, easy to understand guidelines for wellbeing. His own personal story and motivation for improving his health is inspiring."

—Katie Kaps Co-CEO HigherDOSE NYC

Progress Over Perfection

16 Simple Steps to Reclaim Your Health and Wellbeing

Gregg C. Roberts, INHC

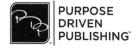

PURPOSE
DRIVEN
PUBLISHING

For permission requests, write to the publisher, addressed "Attention: Permissions Coordinator," at the address below.

Purpose Driven Publishing
141 Weston Street, #155
Hartford, CT 06141

The opinions expressed by the Author are not necessarily those held by Purpose Driven Publishing.

Ordering Information: Quantity sales and special discounts are available on quantity purchases by corporations, associations, and others. For details, contact the publisher at the address above.

Edited by: Heather B. Habelka
Cover design by: Alex Valchev
Interior design by Polgarus Studio

Printed in the United States of America.

ISBN: 978-1-946384-14-0 (print)
ISBN: 978-1-946384-15-7 (ebook)
Library of Congress Control Number: 2017947885

First edition, October 2017.

The information contained within this book is strictly for informational purposes. This publication contains the opinions and ideas of its author. It is intended to provide helpful and informative material on the subjects addressed in the publication. It is sold with the understanding that the author and publisher are not engaged in rendering medical, health or any other kind of personal professional services in the book. The material may include information, products, or services by third parties. As such, the Author and Publisher do not assume responsibility or liability for any third party material or opinions. Readers are advised to do their own due diligence when it comes to making decisions. The author and publisher specifically disclaim all responsibility for any liability, loss or risk, personal or otherwise, which is incurred as a consequence, directly or indirectly, of the use and application of any of the information contained in this book.

For more information visit PurposeDrivenPublishing.com.

Acknowledgements

The older I get the more grateful I have become. In the process of writing this book there are many I feel grateful towards for their contributions, both big and small.

I would like to start by thanking my wonderful publishing team, Jenn T. Grace, Heather B. Habelka, and Niki Gallagher-Garcia at Purpose Driven Publishing for their professionalism, support, and dependability.

Thanks to my mother for her support along the way as well as my three children, Jake, Isabella, and Ava for being involuntary participants in my food and lifestyle exploration journey.

Thank you to Joshua Rosenthal for the wisdom he shares with so many people through his invaluable teaching and the compassionate professionals he surrounds himself with at the Institute for Integrative Nutrition (IIN).

I'd like to thank David Katz for being a champion behind the vital 'lifestyle as medicine' movement and all the hard work he does to spread the message through his various initiatives like the True Health Initiative.

This book took me years to write and along the way there are others who deserve acknowledgement.

Ruth, who helped me get the ideas on paper. Eli for his time and insight. Tami for her support, encouragement, and patience. Michael for sharing his creativity and design talents. Scott for helping me through a roadblock. And Christie, for her special insight and input.

Lastly, I'd like to thank God for His endless mercy, love, and grace.

Dear Reader,

I am absolutely thrilled that you are open to taking *Simple Steps to Reclaim Your Health and Wellbeing.*

This book is meant to supplement rather than replace the advice of your doctor or other trained health professional. Consult with your healthcare practitioner before starting any diet or supplement regimen. The author (me) of this book does not dispense medical advice or other professional advice or prescribe the use of any technique as a form of diagnosis or treatment for any physical, emotional, or medical conditions.

The intent of the author is only to offer information of an anecdotal and general nature that may be part of your quest for emotional, spiritual, and overall wellbeing. All efforts have been made to ensure the accuracy of the information contained in this book as of the date of publication.

The reader (you) should consult his or her medical, health, or other professional before adopting any of the suggestions in this book or drawing inferences from it. This publication contains the opinions and ideas of its author. The author and publisher specifically disclaim all responsibility for any liability, loss or risk, personal or otherwise, which is incurred as a consequence, directly or indirectly, of the use and application of any of the information contained in this book.

You are about to embark on something special. Enjoy!

Gregg C. Roberts

Contents

Foreword by Joshua Rosenthal......................................xiii

Introduction 1

Chapter 1: The Problem 5

Chapter 2: Rocket Fuel..17

Chapter 3: What We See Is NOT What We Get....................29

Chapter 4: If You Don't Like It, Don't Eat It (or Do It)!............43

Chapter 5: Gut Outta Here 49

Chapter 6: Calcium, Carbs, and Other
Nutritional Shades of Gray 65

Chapter 7: Moving On Up 75

Chapter 8: Ree-Lax...81

Chapter 9: Snooze It or Lose It...................................93

Chapter 10: Giving = Living......................................101

Conclusion 107

References...111

About the Author 115

Foreword by Joshua Rosenthal

For over 30 years, I have studied and taught about health, wellness, and nutrition.

It is an interesting field—the only field wherein you can find studies with outcomes that diametrically oppose one another, yet are both proven to be true.

Out of my curiosity and intense studies, I developed a concept called "bio-individuality," basically meaning that what works for one person may not necessarily work for everyone, and vice versa. Essentially, there is no one diet that suits all people.

Furthermore, I realized that health is not all about what you eat. Other aspects of your life will also impact your health—either positively or negatively. I call these "Primary Foods"—things that nourish you that can't be found on your plate. These are things like career, physical activity, relationships, and spirituality. If even one of these areas is incomplete or unfulfilling, your health will be out of balance.

What I've found to be most effective in working with clients is taking a holistic approach to health and wellness. Perhaps the simplest question you can ask a client to determine where their life is out of balance is, "What's missing from your life?" A simple question, but profoundly impactful.

If you're reading this book, it's my guess that you are on a path to a place of better health and wellness. Not only that, but happiness, as joy is an essential component of health.

In the pages of this book, you will find resources, tips, and wisdom for making simple shifts to improve your health and happiness. It does not have to be hard. In fact, most changes you make will be simple yet revolutionary.

Where most people fail in this process is by making too many changes at once, or in overcomplicating the process. Don't do that to yourself.

Instead, follow the steps outlined in this book. Commit yourself to this process of making small shifts to improve your health and wellness. Before you know it, your life will be radically different.

Small changes turn into big changes over time. You just have to have patience with the process.

joshua

—*Joshua Rosenthal, MScEd, Founder and Director, Institute for Integrative Nutrition*

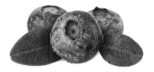

Introduction

"The doctor of the future will be oneself"
—Dr. Albert Schweitzer

We live in a cure-obsessed society that expects a magic pill to arrive on our doorstep—via Amazon Prime—that will keep us healthy, fit, and happy forever. Since most know that day will likely never come, the question becomes, *"What can I do now to take control over my own health and the health of my family?"*

In order to get to the root of this question we must adopt an open mind and do our best to avoid the unnecessary distractions that surround us. The amount of "noise" out there can be overwhelming, particularly when it comes to our health. Whether it is the latest supplement, super food, or elixir promising us eternal health, these well-marketed claims are never-ending. There are more diets than can be counted, and they all promise results. Which one is right? How much sleep do I need? Can I afford to eat well? I have cancer in my family, am I doomed? The list of questions goes on.

This book seeks to answer some of these questions with simple answers and doable action steps.

We live in a cure-obsessed society that expects a magic pill to arrive on our doorstep—via Amazon Prime—that will keep us healthy, fit, and happy forever.

1

℘

My journey to experience my ideal health began around the time of my divorce, which occurred during the tail end of the Great Recession (2008-09). With three young kids (ages ten, five, and three), a marriage that was unraveling, and a demanding professional career in New York City, I had some tough decisions to make. Living in Connecticut and running a company in midtown Manhattan was no longer sustainable for me to be the kind of father I felt my kids needed. So I decided, together with my partners, to close my business.

My health insurance had always been through my wife's employer. She worked for a large airline and had superb health benefits. The day our divorce was finalized, I was officially off the family health insurance plan and for the first time in my life—uninsured. Since their Mom was a flight attendant with an erratic schedule, the kids were often with me more than half the time. One day it hit me that without health insurance and three kids to care for, I simply could not afford to get sick!

As the son of two cancer survivors, with a history of high cholesterol and fluctuating weight, I was highly motivated to do all I could to avoid getting sick. Although I had been involved in the health and fitness business much of my adult life, I had only a rudimentary understanding of real nutrition and wellness. As I began to unpeel the layers of the health and wellness onion, I was blown away by how entirely preventable most chronic illness is. The evidence proving the impact of lifestyle on our overall health and wellbeing was, and is, overwhelming and conclusive.

And yet, we continue to become sicker.

> The evidence proving the impact of lifestyle on our overall health and wellbeing was, and is, overwhelming and conclusive.

According to the Centers for Disease Control and Prevention (CDC), in 2016 life expectancy in the U.S. actually went down for the first time in decades.[1] We spend far more than any other country per capita on health care costs, continue to have exploding chronic illness rates, and mental illness continues to become more prevalent.

Since childhood I'd always believed the old adage, "You are what you eat." My problem growing up and well into adulthood was that I didn't understand *what* I was eating. I didn't know my favorite college meal of boxed mac and cheese or ramen noodles had virtually no nutritional benefit to my body. Although I believed fruits and vegetables were good for me, I didn't understand just how good and important they were, or how much I needed to consume on a daily basis.

Until my own personal journey began, I was unaware of how vital a *balanced lifestyle* was to my overall health. I worked out mostly for vanity up until my thirties and although I knew exercise was good for me, I didn't fully grasp how important it was for my overall health and wellbeing until I was in my early forties.

Same for sleep. I prided myself on being able to get by on four to six hours a night. Today, the evidence supporting the need for at least seven hours is indisputable. Yep, Mom was right all along on this one!

∞

Stress management took a bit longer for me to fully grasp. Some stress is to be expected; it is a natural part of life. And while we cannot always control the situations that bring unwanted stress flooding into our lives, we can control how we manage our *reaction* to stress.

The last area of importance in maintaining overall good health and wellness is mindfulness. While this term has many definitions,

---

[1] http://www.npr.org/sections/health-shots/2016/12/08/504667607/life-expectancy-in-u-s-drops-for-first-time-in-decades-report-finds

there is mounting evidence that those who believe in something outside of themselves generally live healthier lives.

In his book, *The Blue Zones Solutions*, which examines the five communities in the world with the longest lifespans, *National Geographic* journalist Dan Buettner said one of his most surprising findings was the faith factor. He found that 260 of the 265 centenarians (those who live to one hundred years or longer) he had studied included some type of active faith practice in their lives.

₧

My wish, as you begin to read this book, is that you will begin a deeper journey toward greater health and begin to discover the tremendous positive impact lifestyle can have on your wellbeing. My aim is to present the information in as simple and easy a format as possible so you can understand it, implement it, and make it a part of your daily life.

As you move through each chapter, please keep in mind you are unique—a one-size-fits-all approach to health and wellbeing does not work. So what works for your husband or sister may not work for you—and that's okay. I don't expect you to turn your lifestyle upside down overnight. I want you to discover what works best for YOU, in a way and timeframe that works with your lifestyle and wellness goals.

Together, we'll ditch that airbrushed idea of perfection, begin to make small modifications to your existing lifestyle, and do our best to build a life of *lasting* health, wellness, and happiness.

Get ready to add years to your life and life to your years!

Together, we'll ditch that airbrushed idea of perfection, begin to make small modifications to your existing lifestyle, and do our best to build a life of *lasting* health, wellness, and happiness.

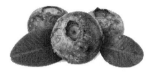

Chapter 1: The Problem

"In all of nature there is no such thing as staying the same. You are either striving to be better or allowing yourself to become worse."
—Unknown

The reality is that most of us treat our cars better than we treat our bodies. We don't fill up with junk fuel, we change the oil, get our periodic tune-ups, and we strive to avoid accidents. Why? Because we know there are unwanted and often expensive consequences to mistreating our cars.

I believe we prioritize our *replaceable* cars over our bodies and minds for one of the following five reasons:

1. Lack of information (we don't know)
2. Apathy (we know, but we don't care)
3. Stagnation (we feel stuck in our daily routine)
4. Feeling Overwhelmed (we don't know how or where to begin)
5. Lack of Self-esteem (we don't think we are deserving)

Do one or more of these reasons resonate with you?

Let's get started on our journey together by looking at some of the cold, hard scientific facts. Trust me, once you've read them, they are impossible to ignore.

Obese & Overweight

Today in the U.S. over 1 in 3 adults is considered obese (BMI of 30+). More than 2 in 3 adults are overweight (BMI of 25+). Additionally, 1 in 20 adults are considered to have extreme obesity (BMI of 40+). About 1 in 3 children ages 6 to 19 are overweight and 1 in 6 children are obese. If you aren't familiar with the term BMI, or Body Mass Index, it is a measure of body fat based on height and weight. Although not a perfect measurement, since it does not distinguish between body fat and lean muscle mass, it is still the most commonly used indicator of obesity.

Prevalence of Obesity among Adults in 2011-2014[2]:

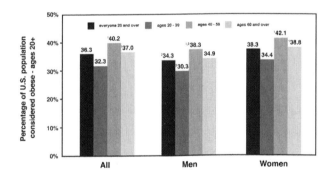

¹Significantly different from those aged 20-39.
²Significantly different from women of the same age group.

NOTES: Totals were aged-adjusted by the direct method to the 2000 U.S. Census population using the age groups 20-39, 40-59,and 60 and over. Crude estimates are 36.5% for all, 34.5% for men, and 38.5% for women.
SOURCE: CDC/NCHS, National Health and Nutrition Examination Survey: 2011-2014

Considering the overwhelming evidence that obesity is a strong precursor for numerous chronic illnesses, it is a staggering fact to

---

² https://www.cdc.gov/nchs/data/databriefs/db219.pdf

consider that such a high rate of obesity currently exists in the U.S.

To describe the situation as an epidemic, particularly among children, would be an understatement.

Diabetes

In 2016, over 40% of the U.S. population was estimated to have diabetes or prediabetes.[3] By 2020 it is estimated that half of all American adults will develop diabetes (or prediabetes). The total annual cost of this care is predicted to be $500 billion by the end of the decade. From 2010 until 2020 we are predicted to spend $3.3 trillion on diabetes care alone. One of the greatest risk factors for diabetes is being overweight.

Cancer

In the 1950s 1 out of 12 people was diagnosed with cancer. Today, close to 1 out of every 2 people is predicted to develop some type of cancer during their lifetime. While more advanced diagnostics may partially explain this increase in cancer rates, it does not account for all of it, meaning that we are clearly moving in the wrong direction despite medical "advances".

Within 20 years, experts are projecting cancer cases to affect 57% of the population.[4]

Does this mean we are destined for a life of sickness? Absolutely not.

---

[3] http://www.unitedhealthgroup.com/newsroom/articles/news/united health%20group/2010/1123whitepaper5usdiabetes.aspx
[4] http://www.cnn.com/2014/02/04/health/who-world-cancer-report/index.html

Does this mean we are destined for a life of sickness? Absolutely not.

My Wake-Up Call

About 10 years ago I was on vacation with my family at a beautiful seaside hotel with a pool overlooking the ocean. In trying to balance my work and family life, I had let myself go. As a kid I was athletic and fit, so I took for granted that staying in good shape was not something I would need to worry about. Judging by my protruding abdomen, love handles, and lack of anything resembling even a "one pack," I was dead wrong. As I was taking in the magnificent ocean vista while treading water (due to my desire to submerge my bloated body underwater and out of sight), I remember feeling a sense of shame that I had allowed myself to fall into such poor shape.

More importantly, back home I noticed I was feeling sluggish. My energy level had declined and fatigue would set in at some point during the course of the day. I was getting at least one case of the cold and flu every year, and my doctor was suggesting medication for my high cholesterol. Where sleep was concerned, I was lucky to get six hours of shut-eye per night. Compounding my unhealthy and unbalanced lifestyle was a faltering marriage which served to exacerbate the stress of trying to juggle my career and family. Sound familiar?

So back at the hotel, I remember sheepishly walking up the underwater steps to leave the pool, feeling like the middle age slob I had never imagined I would turn into. It was at this moment I told myself it was time to make some serious changes in order to lose weight and begin taking better care of myself. Resolving to begin as soon as I returned home from vacation helped to momentarily alleviate my feelings of shame and embarrassment.

Was my newfound vacation inspiration enough to for me to begin a newfound quest for better health? Nope.

My wake-up call came the day my divorce was official. Why? I was no longer covered under my now ex-wife's medical insurance. With no health insurance, no job, and three young children to care for, the realization hit me like a drone missile strike—*I simply could not afford to get sick.*

Since I was no longer tasked with the responsibility of running a business, I had more free time (though limited resources) to pursue a greater understanding of what ideal wellness really looked like. A friend who had successfully battled cancer suggested I read the book *The China Study*—that transformed the way he looked at nutrition and it transformed my career.

I set out to read every book, watch every documentary, and devour every credible article I could get my hands on when it came to health and wellness. I also went back to school to become a certified Integrative Nutrition Health Coach at the Institute for Integrative Nutrition in New York City.

∞

Today I work with companies to improve their health and wellbeing—one team member at a time. It is always very gratifying to witness the personal and community transformation that can happen when an organization makes the wellbeing of their staff a priority and puts a plan into action.

From my training, research, and coaching practice, I've come to believe that we have significant control over our health—that getting older is *not* an automatic sentence for physical pain, monthly dependence on our doctors, a medicine cabinet full of medication, dwindling savings from all of our medical costs, and less overall joy in our lives.

> We have significant control over our health—getting older is *not* an automatic sentence for physical pain, monthly dependence on our doctors, a medicine cabinet full of medication, dwindling savings from all of our medical costs, and less overall joy in our lives.

Grandma Grace

While I was in college I had the good fortune to live with my 90-year-old grandmother, who in hindsight, planted many seeds of wellness wisdom within me. She lived to the ripe old age of 101 and up until her late nineties she shopped for her own food, did calisthenics, gardened, enjoyed a weekly game of bridge, and completed the *LA Times* crossword puzzle daily.

Grandma avoided salt and sugar. In fact, if I were to reach for the saltshaker, which was only laid out on the table for guests, I might get a slap on my hand followed by her patented line, "You don't need any more salt on that Gregg. It has more than enough salt in it already." My grandmother was on to something here.

The Food and Drug Administration (FDA) recommends we limit our daily sodium consumption to 2300 milligrams—about a teaspoon of salt. For those seeking optimum heart health, the American Heart Association (AHA) recommends we should not consume more than 1500 mg per day[5]—less than ¾ of a teaspoon of salt. Why do we need to be concerned about our sodium intake? Lower sodium intake has been associated with a significant reduction in blood pressure, which in turn reduces the risk of heart disease (still the #1 killer in the U.S.) and stroke.

---

[5] https://sodiumbreakup.heart.org/how_much_sodium_should_i_eat

My grandmother was also a stickler for watching her sugar intake, and mine, while I lived with her. She loved to bake but would often use only 1/3 of the sugar the recipe called for. She never hesitated to announce this fact when she baked. Since I was used to sweeter delicacies, I can't say I always loved her baked goods, but over time, I got used to her baking and eventually enjoyed it.

Grandma Grace was sharp. She didn't just dabble in the *LA Times* crossword, she wouldn't rest until every square contained a letter. Despite my being an active college student and English major, she would kick my butt in Scrabble without fail. I was never able to claim even *one* victory (it was during these Scrabble games I first discovered her competitive nature). She also played bridge weekly with a group of friends and would usually emerge victorious.

Her house was situated on the edge of a beautiful hill close to downtown Los Angeles that overlooked the Hollywood Hills. There was a steep drop down off a cliff on the north-facing side of the house. One day I was outside reading in the garden and she was doing some weeding on a small perch that jutted out from this cliff. She obviously did not suffer from a fear of heights.

Suddenly I heard her shouting my name, so I jumped up from my lawn chair to discover a swarm of bumblebees around her. After an initial shortage of courage, I eventually managed to literally drag her up and over the ledge without pulling her then 93-year-old arms out of their sockets.

When we got safely inside the house and assessed the damage, she had what appeared to be a dozen rather large welts all over her arms, shoulders, upper back, and neck. My offer to take her to the doctor was met with complete resistance. It was clear a discussion about the matter would not change her mind so I offered her some aspirin. She turned it down, asked me for a glass of water, and informed me she would sit down as she was feeling "a bit light headed."

Grandma was back outside weeding within an hour.

What did I learn from living with this remarkable woman? At the time, that I needed to sneak salt and hide candy. Today, I have come to appreciate how her simple wisdom has impacted my own wellness journey.

Lessons Learned from Grandma Grace:

Lesson 1. *Don't add more salt to food.* Most food already comes with more than enough salt. It's better to season with herbs.

Lesson 2. *Avoid processed foods.* If we can't pronounce the ingredient, it is best not to consume it. Food is grown to be harvested and eaten—not shelved. Frozen is fine if fresh is not an option.

Lesson 3. *Eat plenty of fresh fruits and vegetables.* Every day without fail she would make sure that both of us consumed several servings of fruits and vegetables. Also, she believed it was better to undercook vegetables so they would retain more nutrients. She was right!

Lesson 4. *Drink lots of water and avoid sweetened drinks.* I have this image in my mind of Grace sitting at the head of the dining table, staring out into the backyard, enjoying a glass of water. I remember wondering if she was even thirsty or drinking just because she felt she needed to.

Lesson 5. *Moderation and portion control.* This lesson was learned more through observation than practice with Grandma. In her eyes, I was her growing grandson with a ravenous appetite so if there were leftovers I was always offered them and I almost always accepted. My wiser grandmother, on the other hand, consumed small portions and would rarely have seconds—other than leftover vegetables. She also detested waste, so she was mindful about not preparing more food than the two of us would need. She also ate a wide variety of most foods and enjoyed homemade desserts as well as occasional red meats—in moderation.

Lesson 6. *MOVE*. Grandma rarely stayed still. Even when she was well into her late nineties she was on her feet and moving most of the time. If she was sitting, it was only to eat, work on her beloved crossword puzzles, read, or play bridge. Every morning she would begin her day with 15 minutes of calisthenics in her bedroom.

Lesson 7. *Don't watch too much TV*. My grandmother had a TV, but outside of an important political debate or major breaking news story, she had little interest in watching television.

Lesson 8. *Get proper rest*. Grandma was a classic example of early to bed, early to rise.

Lesson 9. *Exercise the mind*. Between reading her daily newspapers, crossword puzzles completed to perfection, bridge playing, and active friendships, Grandma kept her brain active and alert.

Lesson 10. *Kindness*. Grandma was kind and cared deeply for those around her. She was always willing to help a friend, family member, or neighbor in need. This kindness was often taken advantage of by the occasional tradesperson or neighbor, but she had a forgiving heart and never held on to any bitterness.

Lesson 11. *Integrity is a must*. My grandmother was as honest and honorable a person as they come. She ALWAYS kept her word.

Telling the absolute truth—regardless of the consequences—was the only option for her.

If you're wondering what the last three lessons have to do with our health and wellness, let me explain. Lesson 9 is easy to clarify since the mind is like a muscle, which should be exercised for optimal performance. There are numerous studies to support the theory that keeping the mind active, especially as we age, helps improve cognition, and can help prevent chronic diseases such as Alzheimer's. Those individuals who continue to stay mentally engaged well into their later years show far fewer signs of mental degeneration than those who do not. Consider Sumner Redstone, who was still working as the Chairman of Viacom and CBS into his nineties. Or Dr. Ellsworth Wareham, from Loma Linda, CA, a cardiovascular surgeon (who happens to be vegan), still performing open-heart surgeries at the age of 98!

According to Paul Pearsall, PhD, and author of the book *The Pleasure Prescription,* "Modern research shows one of the most pleasurable of all human acts is also one of the healthiest things you can do for yourself and for others. Gentle, caring selflessness results in significant health benefits."[6] In essence, *kindness,* Lesson 10, helps sustain healthy lives. Sure, there are some crotchety folks who manage to live past the average lifespan, but these curmudgeons are usually not as healthy or happy as the "kind" crowd.

Integrity, Lesson 11, is not as commonly connected to our longevity, so I will offer my own theory here. We all know the expression "I just want to go to bed at night with a clear conscience." Why? I believe if we have done something wrong or dishonest it bothers us. Not having a clear conscience can disrupt our

---

[6] https://sodiumbreakup.heart.org/how_much_sodium_should_i_eat

concentration and interrupt our sleep.

My grandmother was born in 1898 in a world far different than the one we live in. Today, our food sources are less pure. The food industry manufactures more food-like substances than it provides actual (whole/real) food. And the industry is craftier than ever with their marketing techniques. We lead sedentary lives due to technology and transportation advancements. More prescription drugs are being prescribed per capita now than ever before with a seemingly infinite number of side effects. We have new chronic illnesses, allergies, food sensitivities, and autoimmune disorders popping up every year. Herein lies the problem.

Simple Step #1: Increase your own level of knowledge and insight by watching some entertaining ground-breaking documentaries on health and wellness. A few of my favorites are *Food, Inc., Forks over Knives*, and *Fed Up*.

Progress Over Perfection Action Questions:

1. How do you rate your overall health and wellness? Are you content with your health the way it is? If not, how would you like to improve it?

2. If you were to continue living the same lifestyle that you have now, what do you imagine your health will look like in 20 years?

3. How do you imagine your life would be impacted if you made some small positive changes to your lifestyle such as eating one serving of greens with your dinner and walking 30 minutes each day?

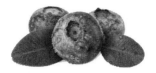

Chapter 2: Rocket Fuel

"Let food be thy medicine and medicine be thy food."
—Hippocrates

Sherri Mraz, a certified integrative nutrition health coach and founder of the Wellness Cooking Academy, offers the following advice to her clients, "Before you eat something, ask yourself whether the food will hurt you or heal you."

The unfortunate reality is that most foods in a typical supermarket are hurting us. In fact, most of what we consume today would not even be considered real food.

The culprit?

"Before you eat something, ask yourself whether the food will hurt you or heal you."

Processed Foods

Most of what we actually consume today are a mixture of chemical ingredients not found in nature combined together to *resemble* food that tastes so good we come back for more. The Oxford Dictionary defines food as "any nutritious substance that people or animals eat or drink, or that plants absorb in order to maintain life and growth." How many foods in your typical supermarket would actually pass the test to qualify as food as Oxford defines it? My estimate? Around 20% at a conventional grocery store. As much as the masterful food manufacturers and marketers may try to give the appearance of their product being food, the undeniable fact is that most of what is boxed and canned is not *real* food.

Why is this so important and how does it actually affect us?

Beside the fact that so many people are unwittingly consuming empty calories from substances that are not actually real food, we now know that the effect of food on genetic expression and cell function is a major cause behind our current epidemic of chronic disease.

> As much as the masterful food manufacturers and marketers may try to give the appearance of their product being food, the undeniable fact is that most of what is boxed and canned is not *real* food.

The Body's Environment

Jing X. Kang, MD, PhD, from Harvard Medical School, and the editor of *The Journal of Nutrigenetics and Nutrigenomics* asserts, "We now understand that a variety of environmental stimuli trigger changes in gene expression, and that these changes underlie disease; for example, a decrease in global DNA methylation can upregulate genes involved in disease, such as cancer-promoting genes, thereby heightening the risk of developing cancer. Clearly, nutrition and diet constitute a major source of environmental input, and there is reason to believe that increases in metabolic disease are associated with recent changes to the human diet and its impact on the genome."[7]

To simplify, Dr. Kang makes the very important connection between nutrition—a major source of our body's environmental stimuli (which is defined as anything existing in the environment that affects humans and other animals or things)—and our risk of disease. So the foods we eat are actually changing the process (gene expression) by which all that valuable information contained within our genes is used or expressed. These *changes* are now understood to be underlying factors for what causes chronic disease like cancer.

∞

The Centers for Disease Control reported that in 2012 about half of all adults in the U.S. had one or more chronic health conditions; 1 in 4 had two or more chronic health conditions; 7 of the top 10 causes of death in 2010 were from chronic diseases; and chronic illness rates are projected to continue to rise steeply.

A study published in the *Journal of the American Medical Association* showed that the rate of chronic health conditions among children in the United States increased from 12.8% in 1994 to 26.6% in 2006.[8] Let's pause for a second on this last statistic. In just 12 short years the chronic illness rates among our country's children more than doubled!

Think Dr. Kang may be on to something?

There is little doubt within the wellness community that much of what is behind the explosion and rising trends of chronic illness is the lack of nutritious foods we are consuming in favor of the processed stuff. What we ingest is so important, that besides the

---

[7] https://www.karger.com/Article/Pdf/339375
[8] http://www.medscape.com/viewarticle/717030

impact it has on our overall health, the foods we choose to eat are triggering changes in our gene expression!

Now this information may seem scary or come across as downright depressing, but the great news is we can choose to eat what our bodies are meant to consume and experience the often tremendous benefits from doing so.

Rocket Fuel

Rocket fuel, as I call them, are foods that that are loaded with all kinds of nutrients, vitamins, and minerals which are commonly referred to as whole foods. It is a long list, but most of what comes from nature and has not been altered, modified, or processed in any way is considered a whole food. Think broccoli, romaine lettuce, spinach, kale, and those other dark leafy greens. Think nuts, legumes like black beans, and tomatoes. Whole grains like oatmeal, brown rice, or quinoa. Avocados and olive oil.

Let's go back to the car metaphor as we begin to examine what's in our pantry, our refrigerator, and our shopping cart. If we put impure or lesser quality gas into our cars what will happen?

We all are familiar with the 87, 89, and 93 octane ratings posted on those yellow buttons every time we buy gas. Most cars operate fine on the minimum 87 octane, but the higher performance cars like a Ferrari or a Lamborghini require 93 octane to perform the way they were built to. According to the Fuel Freedom Foundation operating a car with a gas that is less than an 87 octane rating "and you risk damaging your engine."

Let's imagine applying this principal to the foods we consume. Since we have so much choice, and tend to naturally gravitate to what tastes the best over what is actually nutritious, most of us are eating sub-par, lower than 87-octane food. What are some of the consequences for this? Look no further than the skyrocketing rates of chronic illness.

> **Simple Step #2:** Eat at least one serving of dark leafy green vegetables* per day
>
> *Check with your doctor if you are on any medication as there may be certain vegetables that do not mix well with certain drugs.*

There are several fun food documentaries that demonstrate the transformative effects of putting rocket fuel food in our bodies. In *Fat, Sick and Nearly Dead*, the film's subject, Joe Cross, took himself on a self-guided journey from sickness to health. He was at least 100 pounds overweight, suffering from a debilitating autoimmune disease, and taking a boatload of meds. He wasn't having success with doctors and the conventional medicines being prescribed, so he turned to his own body's ability to heal itself. He decided to try living solely on fresh fruit and vegetable juices for 60 days. The result—he lost 100 pounds, got off the meds, and felt phenomenal. He subsequently cut out the junk food, improved his lifestyle, and continued to eat rocket fuel foods. The transformation was so significant for many who watched the film that a sequel was made—*Fat, Sick and Nearly Dead 2*.

I know this is an extreme example, but stay with me!

Another film that drives the point home about the sheer value of consuming rocket fuel food is *Forks Over Knives*, which is based on 20 years of research published in the book, *The China Study*.

The China Study, written by Cornell University professor T. Colin Campbell and his son Thomas M. Campbell, a medical doctor, was partially based on a collaborative study between Cornell, the University of Oxford, and the Chinese Academy of Preventive Medicine, where Professor Campbell was one of the directors. The *New York Times* called the study "the Grand Prix of epidemiology" for good reason, as it is known to be one of the more credible and comprehensive studies ever conducted in the area of nutrition.

The study looked at mortality rates from cancer and other chronic diseases in 65 counties in China—both rural and urban. The conclusion was that the counties with a high consumption of animal-based foods, like processed meats and dairy, were likely to experience higher death rates from Western diseases, while the opposite was true for counties that ate more plant-based foods. In other words, the people who lived in the counties where they consumed more plant-based foods (rocket fuel) had much lower incidences of chronic illness.

The film *Forks Over Knives* took the findings one step further than *The China Study*. To drive home the strong case for food as medicine, the documentary followed "reality patients" who were suffering from a range of chronic conditions including heart disease and diabetes. Under the supervision of doctors and the scrutiny of the camera, one by one these reality patients were able to shed all or most of their meds, lose weight, experience greatly improved cholesterol levels, and lower their blood pressure. The film helped prove the theory that patients achieved better health after adjusting their eating patterns.

Naturally, all scientific theories can and will be debated, and the field of nutrition is no different. Low fat vs. high fat. Low carb vs. no carb. High protein vs. low protein. Dairy or no dairy. It's never-ending and understandably confusing for most of us. In our individual quest to learn more, we need to experiment with what works best for each one of us, rather than relying on the latest article or (industry funded) study. Avoid striving for perfection and keep it simple and fun.

Speak to any functional doctor, naturopath, or health coach who has witnessed time and again the wonderfully transforming effects of using food and lifestyle as medicine and you will hear more amazing success stories than you can imagine. The evidence of benefits for making these abundant rocket fuel foods the staple of your eating routine is enormous.

For the extra curious check out The Gerson Therapy, a fresh vegetable juice based regimen combined with detox (the process of cleansing or removing poisonous substances/toxins from our body), that has been used over the past 80 years by thousands to successfully treat cancer and other chronic illnesses. The therapy works by "activating the body's extraordinary ability to heal itself"[9]. For the doubtful and more cynical out there, I would encourage you to take the time to do your OWN research. For example, read about some of the patients who had been diagnosed with life threatening illnesses, even cancer, and have had remarkable outcomes after doing Gerson Therapy.

I could take up countless pages here reviewing dietary theory, but my goal is simplicity in order to make this topic as easy to understand as possible. The simple takeaway I want to emphasize is to view whole foods as rocket fuel and question the value of all other food before you make the decision to eat it. The clear advantages to consuming the abundant foods found in nature that can heal, AND taste delicious, are well documented and irrefutable. Mother Nature's food supply is powerful!

> Try to view whole foods as rocket fuel and question the value of all other food before you make the decision to eat it.

---

[9] http://www.Gerson.org

Here's a partial list of rocket fuel foods to help you get started:

Fruit Choices		Vegetable Choices	
Apples	Mango	Artichoke	Garlic
Apricots	Nectarine	Asparagus	Green beans
Blackberries	Orange	Brussels sprouts	Kale
Blueberries	Papaya	Bean sprouts	Kohlrabi
Cantaloupe	Peach	Beets	Leeks
Cherries	Pears	Broccoli	Mushrooms
Dates	Pineapple	Cabbage	Okra
Figs	Plums	Carrots	Onions
Grapefruit	Prunes	Cauliflower	Pea pods
Grapes	Raspberries	Celery	Peppers
Honeydew Melon	Strawberries	Collard greens	Rainbow chard
Kiwi	Tangerines	Cucumber	Romaine Lettuce
Mandarin Oranges	Watermelon	Eggplant	Scallions

As you begin experimenting with the rocket fuel natural foods, notice how your body is feeling. Are you more energized, alert, or lucid? Sleeping better?

Many of my clients report that after incorporating rocket fuel foods into their daily eating habits they notice the adverse effects from overly processed junk foods almost immediately. My client Alan, a CPA and business owner, shared with me the heavy feeling and mild discomfort he experienced from eating pizza after a short period of eating cleaner. This is our body's way of telling us, "C'mon, you've been treating me pretty well here, why are you beating me up with the junk food now?"

Once we start to make whole foods the staple of our nutrition, our bodies begin a natural cleaning process. There are fewer unnatural compounds and toxins for our digestive system to have to process and get rid of. So some of our key organs like the liver, kidneys, and pancreas are no longer working overtime to confront all of the junk compounds and can concentrate more on normal cleansing.

Let's take the liver as an example. Our body's largest organ, the liver is a busy and vital organ responsible for making protein, clotting blood, secreting bile, processing fat, and storing carbohydrates. Brent Tetri, MD, professor of internal medicine at the Saint Louis University Liver Center says, "There's strong evidence now that a fast-food *type* of diet—high in fat and sugar, the kind of diet many Americans subsist on—can cause significant damage to your liver and have extremely serious consequences for your health."[10] He also points out "the good news is that most people can undo this damage if they change their diet and they keep physically active." Good news indeed. Substitute the foods that hurt with the foods that heal.

Substitute the foods that hurt with the foods that heal.

Can I Get a Drink?

What about rocket fuel when it comes to what we drink? This is a very short, simple list:

1. Water. Try adding some slices of lemon or lime for extra flavor.

---

[10] https://www.sciencedaily.com/releases/2008/04/080430204519.htm

2. Fresh-squeezed vegetable juice (a small portion of fruit is okay, but we want to keep an eye on our sugar intake with fresh-squeezed juices)

3. Tea (particularly green)

The jury is out on coffee.

There are many studies from both camps—both pro-java and anti-java. For optimal health benefits, if you choose to drink coffee which does contain antioxidants (nutrients that help prevent tissue damage caused by molecules called oxygen-free radicals which can reduce inflammation, increase immune benefits, and possibly aid in anti-aging effects), I usually suggest fresh brewed lighter roast decaf without milk and sugar. If you enjoy a cup or two of caffeinated coffee throughout the day that is okay, but I would encourage you to experiment with drinking less or cutting out the java for a short time to see how it makes you feel. If you feel less jittery or have more natural energy from eliminating or reducing coffee from your daily routine, you may want to consider cutting it out. If after experimenting with your intake, you don't feel there is any negative effect, go on enjoying in moderation (2-3 cups/day). Remember to be mindful with what you add to your joe. A tasty, healthy alternative is to sprinkle some cinnamon in your coffee.

But before you grab that cup of morning joe, consider green tea which is also loaded with antioxidants plus compounds (and type of antioxidant) called catechins which are highly touted among many nutritional professionals for their ability to fight and prevent cell damage.

Did you know some of those fancy sounding coffee drinks often contain colossal amounts of sugar? Take Starbucks and their Grande Caramel Macchiato with 2% milk, which contains 33 grams of sugar, or Dunkin Donuts medium Mocha Swirl Iced Latte with skim milk, containing 51 grams of sugar in a single serving!

If you opt for plain coffee (0 grams of sugar), even with some whole milk you are looking at only about 2 grams of sugar and only a fraction of the calories.

Christopher Ochner, PhD, research scientist in nutrition at the Icahn School of Medicine at Mount Sinai Hospital in New York City proclaims in no uncertain terms his opinion of green tea, "It's the healthiest thing I can think of to drink."[11] Green tea comes in all types of different flavors and can be enjoyed with some honey and lemon if you prefer.

Give it a try!

Happy Hour?

Unless you struggle with alcohol addiction, consuming alcohol in moderation is usually okay. Moderation is defined by the U.S. Department of Health and Human Services as *up to* 1 drink per day for women and *up to* 2 drinks per day for men.[12] It's important to understand one drink is considered a 12-ounce beer, 5-ounce glass of wine, or a 1.5-ounce serving of 80-proof distilled spirits. We need to be mindful that many of us, along with many restaurants and bars, pour

---

[11] http://www.webmd.com/food-recipes/features/health-benefits-of-green-tea#1
[12] https://www.niaaa.nih.gov/alcohol-health/overview-alcohol-consumption/moderate-binge-drinking

more generously than what is considered to be the standard drink size. It is also important to remember that consuming alcohol will dehydrate us, so be sure to drink extra water while you are enjoying that cocktail.

Simple Step #3: Try drinking an extra glass of water each day with an eventual goal of drinking six to eight glasses per day. An easy first step is to replace one can of soda or fruit juice each day with a bottle of refreshing water. And try adding fresh fruit like lemon, lime, or blueberries to your water—it's delicious!

Progress Over Perfection Action Questions:

1. How would you describe the way you eat and your relationship with food? How much of your food consumption comes from natural, whole sources? How much comes from the drive-thru or is in boxes and cans?

2. Does food make you feel joy or shame? Do you ever find yourself sneaking food out of the sight of others?

3. What is one small step you'll do this week to improve your relationship with food? Are you willing to incorporate one new rocket fuel food per week (or month) into your diet? Are you willing to consider removing one processed food per month from your eating routine?

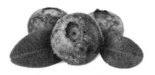

Chapter 3: What We See Is NOT What We Get

"I've grown tired of smoke and mirrors.
I yearn for the clean, well-lighted place."
—Amy Poehler

It is an understatement to say that food marketing can be deceptive. Over 75% of the foods found in a typical American supermarket are not real food, and most are devoid of nutrition. In most cases, the foods we choose are actually doing us more harm than good. The food industry is rife with creating (literally often in a lab) foods by mixing all sorts of ingredients and chemicals together and placing them in beautiful packaging. Often the packaging costs the food manufactures more to make than the actual "food" product!

Take cereal for example. Boxes with friendly looking cartoon characters or handsomely paid celebs touting nutritional claims such as Made with Wholesome, Sweetened Rice Cereal, Good Source of Vitamin D, or Multigrain Cereal Made with Natural Flavors and Colors can be confusing.

There is little to nothing *wholesome* about most sweetened rice cereal. Some of these claims may be partially true (e.g., multigrain cereal), while most patently abuse their use of enticing-sounding adjectives.

Kim Ross, MS, RD, CDN, a respected practicing nutritionist in

New York City has this to say about breakfast cereal, "They are very processed and stripped of the original germ and bran in the way nature intended. All or most of the outer layer of the grain is usually stripped away in the refining process. This means that fiber, vitamins and minerals present in this outer layer are lost. In addition, the grains are often bleached with unwanted chemicals. Although many companies enrich or fortify a cereal with vitamins and/or minerals and even add extra bran, they are rarely in the amounts and ratios present naturally."

Sugar

There is a difference between naturally derived sugar and added sugar. Naturally derived sugars are those that come from fresh fruits, vegetables, and other whole foods. Examples of added sugars are *white sugar, corn syrup, sucrose, dextrose, fructose,* and all artificial sweeteners. These are the sugars that are typically added to processed foods, which many consumers are not even aware of. The American Heart Association recommends no more than 24 grams of added sugars for women and 36 grams of added sugars for men per day.[13] Since few people adhere to the actual manufacturer recommended serving size which the sugar amounts are based on, we often consume far more of what's listed underneath the Nutrition Facts labels, including SUGAR.

For example, if we look at a recommended ¾ cup serving of Kellogg's Frosted Flakes, it contains 12 grams of sugar PLUS another 5.5 grams of sugar for the milk (skim or fat free) for a total of 17.5 grams of sugar. For a woman, that's almost the total

---

[13] http://www.heart.org/HEARTORG/HealthyLiving/HealthyEating/Nutrition/Sugar-101_UCM_306024_Article.jsp#.WVUotIWcFAE

allowable daily intake of sugar of 24 grams—and that's *if* we stay within the recommended serving guidelines. Try measuring out ¾ cup of cereal!

What about Kellogg's Smart Start Strong Heart Antioxidants cereal? That *must* be good for us, right? If we consume the manufacturers recommended 1 cup serving size plus ½ cup of skim milk, we are consuming 19.5 grams of sugar (14 grams from the cereal and 5.5 grams from the milk). Ever wonder why there is a diabetes epidemic in this country?

And it's not just breakfast cereal—sugar is virtually ubiquitous.

Let's take a look at yogurt. We are told yogurt is good for us, especially when fruit is added. If we look at the label of Dannon's Fruit On the Bottom strawberry yogurt there's 24 grams of sugar in one serving! Remember 24 grams of added sugar is the AHA's maximum recommended daily allowance for women. So if you eat one Fruit on the Bottom yogurt, you have already had your daily allowance of added sugar. As an alternative, consider trying plain Greek yogurt, which contains around 6 grams of sugar per serving. Try topping it off with your favorite fruit or a teaspoon of organic honey.

Simple Step #4: For a quick, healthy breakfast, try a whole-grain oatmeal like steel cut oats, topped with your favorite fresh fruit.

As children, many of us grew up eating cereal and yogurt. We were told these choices were good for us.

So what's really going on here? *Added sugar.* It's the dirty secret that the food industry does not want you to figure out. In order to get us coming back for more, our food manufacturers load our foods up with *added* sugar. Take for example the whole misguided low-fat craze that began in the 1970s. Suddenly, and unfortunately as it still continues today, there was a rush by the food industry to concoct foods which contained 'low or no fat.' This was nothing more than removing fat and adding sugar. The food manufactures knew that simply stripping fat from our foods would taste disgusting. So through laboratory experimentation (literally—this is how most of our processed food comes to life) they eventually discovered the secret sauce—JUST ADD MORE SUGAR.

Up until July 2016, the FDA did NOT require food manufacturers to include the percentage of the daily value of sugar and added sugar. Requiring the added sugar disclosure to nutrition labels is certainly a step in the right direction as we decide whether or not to purchase the item for ourselves and our families.

OLD LABEL | NEW LABEL

Nutrition Facts		
Serving Size 2/3 cup (55g)		
Servings Per Container About 8		
Amount Per Serving		
Calories 230	Calories from Fat 72	
		% Daily Value*
Total Fat 8g		**12%**
Saturated Fat 1g		**5%**
Trans Fat 0g		
Cholesterol 0mg		**0%**
Sodium 160mg		**7%**
Total Carbohydrate 37g		**12%**
Dietary Fiber 4g		**16%**
Sugars 1g		
Protein 3g		
Vitamin A		10%
Vitamin C		8%
Calcium		20%
Iron		45%

* Percent Daily Values are based on a 2,000 calorie diet. Your daily value may be higher or lower depending on your calorie needs.

	Calories:	2,000	2,500
Total Fat	Less than	65g	80g
Sat Fat	Less than	20g	25g
Cholesterol	Less than	300mg	300mg
Sodium	Less than	2,400mg	2,400mg
Total Carbohydrate		300g	375g
Dietary Fiber		25g	30g

Nutrition Facts	
8 servings per container	
Serving size	**2/3 cup (55g)**
Amount per serving	
Calories	**230**
	% Daily Value*
Total Fat 8g	**10%**
Saturated Fat 1g	**5%**
Trans Fat 0g	
Cholesterol 0mg	**0%**
Sodium 160mg	**7%**
Total Carbohydrate 37g	**13%**
Dietary Fiber 4g	**14%**
Total Sugars 12g	
Includes 10g Added Sugars	**20%**
Protein 3g	
Vitamin D 2mcg	10%
Calcium 260mg	20%
Iron 8mg	45%
Potassium 235mg	6%

* The % Daily Value (DV) tells you how much a nutrient in a serving of food contributes to a daily diet. 2,000 calories a day is used for general nutrition advice.

https://www.fda.gov/Food/GuidanceRegulation/GuidanceDocuments
RegulatoryInformation/LabelingNutrition/ucm385663.htm

Although still not ideal, the new labels do provide a clearer frame of reference when we are trying to assess how much sugar and added sugar the particular food item contains. (It's important to note that the Food and Drug Administration's guidelines and the American Heart Association's guidelines do not line up. Despite some of their questionable industry relationships and funding sources, I would nevertheless strongly urge you to adhere to the AHA's recommendations over the FDA's since it is widely known that the FDA has multiple food industry relationships and their policies are often influenced by them).

The Great Gluten Debate

You may be wondering about bread and pasta. Unlike cereals and most yogurts, I do eat bread and pasta—in moderation. The key here is to choose wisely. The simplest way to avoid consuming the harmful type is to look at the label. When you start seeing too many multi-syllabic ingredients that you can't pronounce, like Calcium Propionate (an antifungal used as a preservative) or Azodicarbonamide (typically used in food to bleach or whiten flour and also found in yoga mats and sneaker soles) it's best to avoid altogether.

Let's compare two different breads side by side:

Kroger 100% Whole Grain Bread, High Fiber:

whole wheat flour, water, wheat gluten, sugar, whole rye flour, brown rice meal, whole barley flour, whole millet flour, contains 2% or less of: honey, polydextrose, soybean oil, raisin juice concentrate, molasses, salt, calcium sulfate, whole triticale flour, yeast, whole grain oats, oat bran, inulin (chicory root fiber), oat fiber, vinegar, soy flour, sodium stearoyl lactylate, ethoxylated mono- and diglycerides, calcium propionate, ammonium sulfate, azodicarbonamide, monocalcium phosphate, enzymes, guar gum, ascorbic acid.

Ezekial 4:9 Sprouted Whole Grain Bread:

Organic Sprouted Wheat, Filtered Water, Organic Sprouted Barley, Organic Sprouted Millet, Organic Malted Barley, Organic Sprouted Lentils, Organic Sprouted Soybeans, Organic Sprouted Spelt, Fresh Yeast, Organic Wheat Gluten, Sea Salt.

In the case of Kroger's 100% Whole Grain Bread, the third and fourth ingredients listed are wheat gluten and sugar. Although wheat gluten may not be as bad as some critics proclaim, the fact of the matter is that nearly 20 million Americans say they regularly experience stomach problems after eating products that contain gluten[14] which has been linked to celiac disease (Gluten helps create a bond which gives bread its chewy texture and ensures the dough sticks together. It also traps carbon dioxide, which as it ferments, adds volume to the loaf.) Gluten has been around for thousands of years which begs an important question: *If gluten, found in a staple food like bread, has sustained humankind for so long, why has it suddenly become so threatening to our health?* The answer lies in the bread we consume now compared to the bread our parents and ancestors consumed. The version of wheat we consume today is a product of genetic research. Primarily due to industrialization and over farming of the soil we simply cannot easily obtain the purer forms of wheat that were grown 50 or 100 years ago.

Historically, bread was made with three to four ingredients—

---

[14] http://www.newyorker.com/magazine/2014/11/03/grain

typically flour (fresh milled from the wheat's whole kernel), water, yeast, and salt. Because bread was made for consumption and not storage it had a one to two-day shelf life.

The breads manufactured today are designed like many other foods for maximum shelf life (up to five to seven days) at the expense of its nutritional content. This usually means processing flours by removing the bran and the germ where 70% of its nutrients are found. The all-purpose flours commonly used today are usually bleached with either benzoyl peroxide (the same stuff used in acne creams) or chlorine gas. Besides being banned in Europe and other countries, these whiteners and shelf life extending ingredients are believed to be linked with a variety of possible health hazards including liver problems.[15]

So the takeaway: buyer beware when it comes to breads. Avoid most commercial brands with unrecognizable ingredients in favor of homemade, bakery breads, or select organic store brands with *whole grains* and no artificial preservatives. Don't let the sound of baking bread intimidate you. It is much simpler to do then it may sound and there are bread makers that make it even easier! Just be sure to use a high quality whole grain flour such as coconut, buckwheat, or whole wheat.

GLUTEN

Dr. David Perlmutter, a neurologist based in Naples, FL, believes, "As many as 40% of us can't properly process gluten, and the remaining 60% could be in harms way." On the other side of the equation is Donald Karsada, PhD, a researcher at the U.S.

---

[15] http://naturallysavvy.com/eat/scary-ingredients-used-in-bread-manufacturing

Department of Agriculture who says he has found no evidence that a change in wheat-breeding practices might have led to an increase in the incidence of celiac disease. According to Mr. Karsada, "My survey of protein (gluten) content in wheat in the U.S. over approximately the past 100 years did not support such an increase on the basis of historical data in comparison with recent data."[16]

What's the takeaway? Another example of mixed opinions in the field of nutrition. I prefer to err on the side of caution and on real-world observation. Or speak to virtually any functional doctor, a growing class of doctors who focus on the root cause of our illness and commonly treat patients by eliminating certain food groups. One of the food groups these doctors eliminate first is wheat. I am not 100% gluten free. You might catch me indulging in a bread basket while dining out—especially if it's just out of the oven! I subscribe to the school of thought that it is okay (and I actually encourage my clients if there appears to be excessive rigidity) to have their favorite treats once in a while. Try this the next time you eat bread or pasta—observe how it makes you feel afterwards.

Fortunately, and I hear this from just about all of my clients who have begun to reduce the more harmful foods from their diets like the white breads and pastas, is that their intense cravings for the carbs and the sweets gradually begin to disappear. In fact what tends to happen is that the cravings for healthy food actually begin to increase.

As a bona fide sugar addict I was no stranger to ripping through half a box of cookies, a pint of ice cream, or a dozen peanut butter cups. For years, every night around 10 p.m. I would get the most intense craving for sweets that seemed unconquerable. I would guiltily slink into the kitchen to scour the

---

[16] http://www.newyorker.com/magazine/2014/11/03/grain

cupboards for anything sweet. The more I consumed the more shame I would feel.

Curbing my sugar addiction was certainly no overnight affair. It happened gradually when I made a conscious effort to treat my body better. When I began to eat more of the good foods I noticed my cravings for the junk started to wane. Not that I still didn't love a half-pint of cookie dough ice cream, it was just that I began to crave more vegetables and other whole foods. There used to be a restaurant across the street from my former office. I would go up to the bar in the middle of the day and order sautéed spinach with garlic to satisfy my cravings for greens. Once in a while I would get the Popeye quips from the bartender. It was interesting to see how the sugar cravings gave way to my body naturally seeking the foods that were good for me. It's wondrous how our body works. Give it junk, it wants more junk. Give it rocket fuel, it wants more rocket fuel!

Simple Step #5: When you get that midday or late night craving for sweets, try grabbing a piece of fruit or some organic popcorn. Over time you will train your brain and gut out of the intense craving for processed sweets (hurting foods) in favor of seeking the healthier stuff (healing foods). Not easy or natural at first, but it does get easier over time. Be patient with yourself!

The Food Babe

A popular warrior in the fight for food transparency is Vani Hari, also known as the Food Babe. Her before and after story is another transformational success case. As a young, professional woman she suffered from eczema, asthma, allergies, and stomach aches. She was told her conditions were probably genetic, and therefore permanent. She gained a significant amount of weight and landed in the hospital with appendicitis. She then set out to better understand and research health and nutrition. Discovering that most of the food she had been eating was processed with little to no nutrients, she began to develop healthy eating habits.

After initially being turned off by her nom de plume ("Food Babe" didn't resonate with me), at first I heard her speak and was completely sold by her passion and credibility. She and her army of followers are true change agents. They have convinced many well-known restaurant chains and food manufactures to stop using possibly harmful ingredients.

Some of her success stories include:

- Chipotle eventually agreeing to disclose all its ingredients including GMOs (which they now have committed to stop serving entirely)
- Kraft finally agreeing to remove potentially harmful food dyes from their mac and cheese
- Subway consenting to remove a potentially harmful chemical—azodicarbonamide (used in yoga mats and shoe rubber) from their bread
- Panera Bread responding to concerns over some of their ingredients and pledged to remove all artificial colors, flavors, sweeteners, and preservatives

Hari's courageous efforts to expose potentially harmful ingredients in our food sources is just the beginning of developing our food acumen. It is vital we develop a better understanding of exactly what is in the food we eat.

Unfortunately we cannot rely on the Food and Drug

Administration alone to ensure our safety. For example, the FDA refuses to ban the practice of regularly feeding antibiotics to animals that are not sick DESPITE the FDA's own findings that such misuse of antibiotics threatens the effectiveness of essential medicines (not to mention all the possible unknown adverse effects to the people consuming the livestock forced to take these antibiotics). This controversial matter made it all the way up to the Second Court of Appeals in July of 2014 where it ruled in favor of the FDA's position. In a 2-1 decision, the dissenting Judge, Robert Katzmann said, "Today's decision allows the FDA to openly declare that a particular animal drug is unsafe, but then refuse to withdraw approval of that drug. It also gives the agency discretion to effectively ignore a public petition asking it to withdraw approval from an unsafe drug."

In other words, the latest ruling means that even when the FDA is *aware of an unsafe drug,* they do NOT have to withdraw its approval permitting the drug to be fed to livestock that U.S. residents will then be consuming. Farmers are still allowed to use these drugs on the livestock the general public eventually will be eating. It's no surprise to discover current and former FDA commissioners' strong ties to both the pharmaceutical industry and the agricultural industry. For example, Robert M. Califf was both an FDA commissioner and a former lobbyist for multiple large pharmaceutical companies. Michael R. Taylor was also an FDA commissioner as well as a former VP at Monsanto, a large multinational agricultural and agrochemical corporation. Might the fox be guarding the henhouse?

The "Red" Flag

One of the reasons many wellness professionals avoid meat is because of the challenges in ensuring the quality of the meat is safe.

Many of us don't have the time or money to buy meat that was raised and fed properly. It's crazy to think we have to spend so much *more* just to buy meat from cattle or chicken that are grass fed and free range. Just 50 years ago this was how most of our meat and poultry came to us, before the mass production of animal farming became commonplace. The risk of consuming meats that are factory raised is that the animals are not being fed the foods they were meant to eat. In an article in *Mother Jones*, investigative journalist Alex Park discovered that it is not uncommon for cows to be fed sawdust, candy, chicken feces, limestone, and crab guts.[17] If you're like me and believe the expression "you are what you eat", then maybe we should think twice about consuming these types of meats on a regular basis.

Simple Step #6: If you are buying food that comes in a box or a bag, begin to look at the nutritional labels more carefully. There are some helpful apps like Fooducate with bar code scanning features. This app will independently rate each food product with a simple school grade scoring system of A-F for its overall nutritional value, and also let you know if the food contains GMOs.

GMO stands for Genetically Modified Organism. A GMO is an organism (such as food) that has had its DNA altered or modified in some way through genetic engineering. One example is seedless watermelon. Another is a type of goat milk that comes from goats who had a gene from a spider inserted into their DNA to produce silk protein in their goat milk. Currently, food manufacturers are not legally required to disclose GMOs on food packaging. Reading

---

[17] http://www.motherjones.com/food/2013/12/cow-feed-chicken-poop-candy-sawdust/

labels may seem tedious at first, but try having fun with it and look at it as food education that you will be able to share with your loved ones. Another option is to opt for foods that are whole and therefore label reading is unnecessary because there is only one ingredient—the food itself. When was the last time you saw a nutrition label in the produce section of your local grocery store?

Progress Over Perfection Action Questions:

1. How much thought do you give to the food you eat and prepare for your family? Do you consider the source: whole vs. refined foods; organic vs. non-organic; or pasture vs. cage raised? When you eat at a restaurant do you ever wonder what type of ingredients they use?

2. If you knew that certain foods are harmful to your health would you stop eating them? Why or why not? If you were to discover that many foods could help improve your overall health, give you more energy, and strengthen your immune system, would you be motivated to begin including more of these foods into your meals?

3. Currently, what percentage of what you eat would be considered whole foods (foods in their natural state that have not been refined or processed) and what percentage is processed? Would you consider trying to slowly increase the percentage of whole foods you eat if you thought it would improve your overall health and wellbeing?

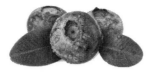

Chapter 4: If You Don't Like It, Don't Eat It (or Do It)!

"Knowledge is knowing a tomato is a fruit.
Wisdom is knowing not to put it in a fruit salad."
—Brian O'Driscoll

One of the first things I do when working with a new client is take an inventory of what they are currently eating, as well as what they ate as a child. My goal is to encourage them to incorporate more healing rocket fuel foods into their meals and begin to gradually reduce the food-like substances that are hurting them.

Since the primary goal for everyone I work with is a *sustainable* healthy lifestyle, ensuring that healthy eating habits continue over time is paramount for overall success. In my experience trying to push foods on people that they do not like is a recipe for failure. Sure, I wish all my clients ate kale, but the truth is not everyone likes kale—and this is okay. There are plenty of other delicious vegetables out there, like sautéed broccoli or a fresh garden salad.

A client and I were reviewing his eating habits on his intake form. It became apparent that he was consuming no healthy foods whatsoever. Fast food and microwaved meals comprised his nutrition. Now, I have worked with some folks who had poor nutrition, but this guy took the cake, literally. I kept scanning his intake form to see if I may have missed something—searching for at least one bit of real food he regularly consumed that would be considered good for him. Nothing. Despite my optimistic tendencies, I was beginning to feel slightly skeptical of this client's prospects. I questioned him to see if he had forgotten to include anything. Finally I asked him flat out, "Hey, I can't help but notice you don't eat any vegetables or fruits. Is this because you don't like the taste? Are there any vegetables that you enjoy eating?" He instantly replied, "I actually love salads!" There was a good chance he noticed the great sense of relief I wasn't able to conceal on my face, "So if I were to ask you to incorporate salads back in to your daily routine this would not be a problem?" "Not at all", he replied. "I can start tomorrow." This small step began a journey that resulted in my client losing 35 pounds within a few months. Today, 18 months later, the weight is still off.

The point here, in the beginning of our wellness journey, is to focus on those foods that are good for us AND that we enjoy eating. One of the many reasons fad diets have failed us over the years is that often they force us to eat food that we dislike and are overly rigid. There are so many wholesome food choices for us to enjoy. If eating starts to feel like an unpleasant task, such as cleaning out our closets or doing our taxes, the chance of long-term success greatly diminishes. It is wise to also recognize the importance of being open to trying new (whole) foods OR foods we haven't had since we were a child that we *think* we don't like. My family will still tease me for not liking lobster as a kid despite our having a summer home on an island off the coast of Maine. I wouldn't touch the stuff. Now, although I don't eat it often, I love lobster.

> You should focus on foods that are good for you AND that you enjoy eating.

> **Simple Step #7:** Remember **A.B.T.** Always **B**e **T**rying. There are hundreds of healthy and delicious whole foods out there. A.B.T. includes trying new supermarkets and farmer's markets as well. The next time you are at the market, pick up a whole food you've never tried before, or something that you haven't had since you were a kid. Variety *is* the spice of life!

Got Resistance?

If we are making the choice to eat a new food or try different types of physical activity, the chances of this behavior sticking are greater than if someone else forces it on us. For example, when it comes to our children, if we force them to play a sport or an instrument that they did not choose, it is unlikely they will thrive over time. If I suggest to a female client who prefers to be outside that she lift weights, fat chance she will still be at the gym in a couple of months. If it turns out this same client prefers cycling, this is where she will enjoy the most long-term success.

And speaking of physical activity, the same principle applies here as well—if you don't like it, don't do it. In fact, I have found with my clients that there is more resistance to certain exercises than to trying new food. Why? Physical activity represents a greater investment of time and often can be more intimidating, at least in the beginning. Most physical activity requires getting out of the house. It may require joining a gym or a health club. There often is additional cost involved. Getting ourselves to the point where we find something we actually enjoy is crucial in order to sustain our routine and good health.

I reached a point years ago when I was tired of lifting weights in a gym. The experience was beginning to feel like drudgery to me. A friend who had just moved to town introduced me to a boxing workout. In the beginning, and because I had never done it before, I was slightly intimidated. But when I finally agreed to try it, I fell in love with the workout! So much that I ended up starting a boxing club for beginners! One of the reasons the club developed a dedicated following was that our customers truly enjoyed the workout. Not only were they getting physical benefits from the workout, they were learning a new skill and having fun at the same time. Men and women alike came to escape the drudgery of the conventional gym experience.

Choose a physical activity you think you might like and give it a try!

Choose a physical activity you think you might like and give it a try!

છ

Initially any change to our routine can be intimidating. This is perfectly natural and should not bring about any shame or guilt. We want to try to break through this barrier of resistance by using strategies that will work for us. For some, a love-based approach works best. We may feel like we deserve to love ourselves more by treating our body better. Or we may have kids/grandkids that we want to enjoy and be active with. For others, fear is the great motivator. One of my clients found out during a routine physical that his triglycerides were 530 when the acceptable upper limit is 150! With a history of heart disease in his family, he and his wife were wisely scared enough for him to immediately seek out health coaching services.

Focus on the "healthy" that appeals to you. As important as it is for us to embrace the necessary changes in our lives that will positively impact our wellbeing, forcing ourselves to undertake diets and exercise regimens that are entirely off-putting is also not the answer. Take those small steps toward progress over unsustainable perfection. Enjoy a cheat day once in a while without shame! *Slow and steady wins this race.*

Progress Over Perfection Action Questions:

1. What do think holds you back from making improvements to your health?

2. How does resistance to potentially positive change show up in other areas of your life?

3. When was the last time you tried a new food or fitness activity? What is one new food you could try this week?

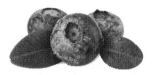

Chapter 5: Gut Outta Here

"All of life is a constant education."

—*Eleanor Roosevelt*

In the Far East it has long been thought that the *root of all illness* comes from the gut which is comprised primarily of the small and large intestine. The father of medicine himself, Hippocrates, also believed this to be true—"All diseases begin in the gut."

This concept is finally being studied more seriously here in the West. Leaky Gut Syndrome, as the condition has come to be known, results from a disproportionate amount of good versus bad bacteria found in our intestines. Our intestines contain a complex community of microbiota, collectively referred to as our microbiome, that lives in the digestive tracts of humans and other animals. These internal gastro environments should contain a ratio of bacteria which is: 80% good to 20% bad. When our guts are not maintaining our proper ratios of microbiota, problems will arise— just like our car's radiator which should have a 50/50 ratio of coolant to water. What happens when we have too much coolant or too much water in our cars? Overheating or frozen radiators, which can lead to far more serious problems. For those of us who like to cook, think about what happens when we get the water to rice ratio reversed. A 1:2 water/rice ratio instead of 2:1 will result in some rice that may not pass many taste tests.

To break it down, when our guts are not maintaining the 80/20 ratio, and begin to approach an imbalance with the bad bacteria tipping the scales at over 50%, this pathogenic (bad) bacteria begins to prevent the healthy gut bacteria from keeping our intestinal lining strong. This imbalance of normal bacteria (flora) is known as dysbacteriosis.

When our intestinal lining is no longer adequately strong, it becomes highly susceptible to damage. It starts with inflammation, and over time, the mucosal lining is destroyed, creating ulcers. This resulting damage begins to allow disease-causing bacteria, toxins, and undigested food particles to pass directly into our bloodstream, where they disrupt our body's normal function in numerous ways.

Is Your Gut Under Attack?

Imagine a castle surrounded by a determined enemy—think *Game of Thrones* or the film *Braveheart*. A well-fortified castle was rarely penetrated instantaneously. The enemy would first locate the most vulnerable point of entry, often the wooden front door which would be covered by a drawn wooden drawbridge. The attacker would usually use a battering ram to break down the door over time. Despite occasional interruptions from the defenders of the castle which could include shooting arrows, setting the battering ram on fire, or pouring hot oil down on the attackers, with persistent battering over time the doors, gates, and drawbridge would eventually be worn down and holes would finally appear within the castle. With some more battering these holes would finally become large enough to enable the attackers to enter the castle and destroy it.

Just as a medieval castle was built to be a strong fortress able to ward off most attacks, so is our gut. In fact, the gut wall has *four layers* of protection—the serous, the muscular layer, the submucosa, and the mucosa. This remarkably designed barrier of our gut is there largely to protect the harmful bacteria and toxins from passing through our intestinal wall and entering our bloodstream. What happens over time when we have an imbalance of good versus bad bacteria within this environment is that the bad flora will begin to wear down these layers of gut protection—much like a battering ram does to a castle. Over time the bad bacteria becomes persistent, attacking and entering our bloodstream. If not stopped, these invaders begins to wreak havoc on our vital organs.

How do we stop the enemy? The answer is simple. Cut out the processed foods, eat more whole foods, and consume more foods rich with probiotics such as unsweetened Greek yogurt, kefir, and fermented foods like sauerkraut, kimchi or dill pickles (Probiotics work to replace the bad bacteria with the good bacteria in our guts. Essentially they are live bacteria and yeasts that are good for our health.) The term "probiotic" did not come into common use until after 1980 and the concept is generally attributed to Nobel Award recipient Elie Metchnikoff. Metchnikoff studied yogurt consuming Bulgarian peasants and found that they lived longer than their counterparts because of this custom.

Simple Step #8: Eat Greek yogurt or kefir, one of the best forms of probiotic foods that is packed with protein. Always opt for the organic, unsweetened variety—you can add fresh fruit or honey for flavor. AVOID low fat and non-fat yogurt (because these usually contain added sugar to compensate for the reduced fat). If you choose to avoid dairy, try affordable, fermented food like pickles, sauerkraut, or kimchi.

For those of you who prefer to get your probiotics in supplement form be sure to adhere to these four rules of thumb when considering your purchase:

1. **High CFU (Colony Forming Unit) Count.** Look for a formula with a minimum of 40 billion CFUs.
2. **The Substrains are Listed.** The substrains listed next to each strain indicates that a specific probiotic strain has undergone clinical studies.
3. **It Contains Prebiotics.** Prebiotics help the probiotics populate and flourish in your gut increasing the overall effectiveness of the probiotic.
4. **The Supplement was Formulated by a Doctor.** Precise formulation and expertise are vital to ensure a more effective supplement.

A less simple, but important tip toward a healthy gut, is to avoid most processed foods. The vast majority of wellness professionals and nutritionists lament the harm caused by the sheer abundance of processed foods in today's food supply. They wreak havoc on our guts and our health.

Most processed foods wreak havoc on our guts and our health.

What exactly are processed foods?

Currently comprising over 70% of the U.S. diet, processed foods are foods that have been altered from their natural state. This is done to increase the shelf life of the food allowing food manufactures and supermarkets to maximize profits, save on shipping costs, and help ensure less costly spoilage—as well as appeal to consumers looking for later expiration dates. It also allows for more marketing opportunities, since packaging provides ample advertising space. The food industry, especially when it comes to dairy, will claim that food safety is a primary reason behind processed foods. They will often point to milk and the pasteurization process as an example of safety in food processing—despite all the evidence out there that shows the risks of pasteurization to our health. Pasteurization is a process of heating a liquid or a food to kill bad bacteria to make the food "safer" to eat. However, the problem with pasteurization is that the process also kills all the good bacteria (probiotics) that our bodies need and damages the vitamins, minerals, and proteins that were originally in the food or liquid.

There are over 5,000 different additives that are allowed to go into our food. The Food and Drug Administration is not able to adequately track which additives are in all of the food we consume. This is partly because regulations are self-regulatory (the food industry itself is doing the testing), and the testing is also often voluntary. Many of these allowable additives such as food dyes[18] and MSG[19] (monosodium glutamate, a flavor enhancer) have been shown to be harmful in numerous lab studies on mice and other animals.

Pros & Cons of Frozen and Canned Foods

One important distinction within the world of processed food is frozen and canned foods. Foods that have been frozen or canned are technically considered (minimally) processed, since they have gone through the process of freezing and canning. These minimally

---

[18] https://cspinet.org/resource/food-dyes-rainbow-risks
[19] http://healthpsych.psy.vanderbilt.edu/HealthPsych/msg.htm

processed varieties are NOT necessarily the processed foods we need to avoid. Organic frozen broccoli for example, is considered processed, although it is still perfectly healthy to consume. In fact, although fresh produce is usually preferable because it contains more active nutrients, most frozen fruits and vegetables are a wise choice when it comes to purchasing reasonably priced produce. Easy to store with a long storage capacity, consuming organic, frozen produce is a perfectly acceptable option when fresh is not readily available, or when shopping on a budget.

Canned, on the other hand, requires more discernment. The producers of canned fruits and vegetables normally cook the produce before packing to ensure there will be no bacterial growth inside the can. This extra cooking destroys nutrients leaving us less by the time we re-cook and consume (every time produce is cooked, some of the nutrients are destroyed). In addition, salt, sugar, artificial sweeteners, and other preservatives are normally added to help better preserve the produce and add flavor. There is also evidence to suggest that harmful chemicals from the cans may seep into our food. Personally, when it comes to canned food, I try to avoid it, with the *exception* of legumes (e.g. black beans, fava beans, chick peas, and kidney beans). When buying canned be sure to read the label carefully. If the list of ingredients contains anything other than sea salt, water, or olive oil, the can will probably not end up in my shopping cart.

Easy to store with a long storage capacity, consuming organic, frozen produce is a perfectly acceptable option when fresh is not readily available, or when shopping on a budget.

According to Livestrong.com, multiple studies indicate that avoiding processed foods leads to lowered blood pressure, reduced weight, improved heart health, and reduced asthma attacks.[20]

> **Simple Step #9:** Avoid processed food whenever possible except minimally processed frozen produce, some canned produce, and wild caught fish such as sardines, tuna, and salmon.

What Are Whole Foods and Why Are They So Important?

Whole foods, such as fruits, vegetables, grains, meats, and non-pasteurized dairy are simply foods that can be consumed in their natural state. Whole foods have not been altered chemically or genetically modified in any way. With most foods, it is obvious what is a whole food, particularly when it comes to fruits or vegetables. Grains and some meat products, however, require further explanation.

Rice

Brown rice is an example of a grain that is considered a whole food. It is whole grain rice, with only the inedible outer hull removed. White rice on the other hand is NOT a whole food since it has the bran layer and cereal germ removed. We should always opt for brown, black, or wild rice which are all whole food varieties that have not been modified in any way and contain the highest amounts of vitamins, minerals, fiber, and other beneficial nutrients.

---

[20] http://www.livestrong.com/article/345172-the-best-non-fattening-snack-foods/

Meat

When it comes to meat, the gauge for its processing can be less transparent. Meats that are grown and sold close to their original state are considered a whole food or minimally processed. Think wild caught fish, grass-fed cattle, and free-range chicken which are simply cleaned, cut, and packaged.

Examples of processed meats are bacon, salami, sausages, beef jerky, hot dogs, and ham which have all gone through multiple steps of processing and contain many added ingredients. Most canned fish options like sardines, tuna, or salmon would be considered minimally processed. So long as there are no unhealthy additives, besides oil (ideally olive or sunflower), water, and salt, some of these canned meats contain nutrients such as protein or omega 3s, and do not necessarily need to be avoided.

Where the processed debate can get more mercurial is around the feeding and living conditions of the animal raised for human consumption. Many in the wellness community, myself included, argue that when the animal is raised in unnatural living conditions such as chickens raised in cages, farm raised fish, or corn fed cattle raised on feedlots, there is a form of processing taking place before they are even slaughtered or caught.

These animals are not being raised in their natural habitats and in the case of most industrialized livestock farms, the animals are being fed an unnatural corn GMO-based feed and given antibiotics. Remember it is not only important which meats WE eat, but also what the animal we are eating *ate*. One of the reasons many more informed people are buying organic meats is to ensure that the meats they are consuming are as close to their natural state as possible and free from unnatural diets, potentially harmful chemicals, and poor living conditions.

> Remember it is not only important which meats WE eat, but also what the animal we are eating *ate*.

Size Matters

In the U.S. we have a serious portion control problem. Nowhere else in the world consumes the types of portions we do (and nowhere else in the world has such a runaway chronic illness problem!) In Asia, a single 6-ounce portion of steak would typically be divided amongst a family of four. Here in the U.S., most restaurants usually serve a *minimum* portion of 10 ounces to a single person. At a backyard BBQ cookout, the average size is similar and can often tip the scales at over 14 ounces.

Here are nutrition labels comparing a 10-ounce steak and a 10-ounce serving of salmon:

Boneless Steak | Wild Caught Salmon

Nutrition Facts

Serving Size: 10 oz, of boneless steak, cooked

Amount Per Serving

Calories from Fat 383
Calories 714

	% Daily Values*
Total Fat 42.55g	65%
Saturated Fat 16.661g	83%
Polyunsaturated Fat 1.585g	
Monounsaturated Fat 17.803g	
Cholesterol 232mg	77%
Sodium 1057mg	44%
Potassium 865mg	
Total Carbohydrates 0g	0%
Dietary Fiber 0g	0%
Sugars -	
Protein 77.37g	

Vitamin A 0%	Vitamin C 0%
Calcium 4%	Iron 30%

* Percent Daily Values are based on a 2000 calorie diet. Your daily values may be higher or lower depending on your calorie needs.

Nutrition Facts

Serving Size: 10 oz, wild caught salmon

Amount Per Serving

Calories from Fat 162
Calories 402

	% Daily Values*
Total Fat 17.96g	28%
Saturated Fat 2.78g	14%
Polyunsaturated Fat 7.194g	
Monounsaturated Fat 5.958g	
Cholesterol 156mg	52%
Sodium 125mg	5%
Potassium 1388mg	
Total Carbohydrates 0g	0%
Dietary Fiber 0g	0%
Sugars -	
Protein 56.21g	

Vitamin A 2%	Vitamin C 0%
Calcium 3%	Iron 13%

* Percent Daily Values are based on a 2000 calorie diet. Your daily values may be higher or lower depending on your calorie needs.

As you can see, one 10-ounce portion of steak is 714 calories before any sauces are added, and contains 65% of our recommended total fat intake, including 83% of our total saturated fat. To many, the more serious nutritional content to consider here is the total cholesterol and sodium. This one 10-ounce portion, considered by many here in the U.S. to be a modest serving of steak, contains 77% of our total cholesterol and 44% of our total sodium *before* we even add salt for taste.

If you are one who chooses to eat steak, consider eating a portion similar to what most of the rest of the world eats which falls into the 3 to 6 ounce range.

If animal protein comprises a significant part of your diet, compare the nutritional content of the same 10-ounce portion of salmon.

Notice the differences in virtually every one of the higher risk areas. The same portion of salmon contains a fraction of the saturated fat, cholesterol, and sodium of its red meat counterpart.

Which choice do you think puts us at higher risk for heart disease? Which source provides us with better overall nutritional value?

I have struggled myself in the portion control department and can still fall prey to overconsumption once in a while. Blame it on a ravenous appetite as a child or parents that allowed me to go back too often for seconds or thirds, but I often find myself lacking an *off* button. Over time, especially since I've focused on consuming more whole foods and cutting way down on my animal protein intake, my appetite has become curtailed and I have a better handle on my portion control. This does NOT mean I am perfect though; I am still known to put quite the dent into a dessert platter around the holidays!

Organic vs. Non-Organic (Conventional)

There is still understandable confusion around the term "organic." What exactly is it? Is it worth the extra cost? Does organic always mean the food is healthy?

My kids used to say, "Dad, we don't like organic. It tastes gross." My kids falsely believed healthy food is tasteless. The truth of the matter is there is no difference in taste between organic and conventionally grown food. It is the same food, except when it comes to the use of pesticides. Non-organic, or conventionally grown foods, typically use pesticides (to kill or repel pests) and herbicides (to destroy weeds and other unwanted vegetation) to keep the insects from eating the crops. Organically grown produce is usually free from such potentially harmful substances.

This is important because many studies show the dangers of humans consuming pesticides over time. The World Health Organization states that "pesticides are potentially toxic to humans and that they may induce adverse health effects including cancer, effects on reproduction, immune, or nervous systems."[21]

> The World Health Organization states that "pesticides are potentially toxic to humans and that they may induce adverse health effects including cancer, effects on reproduction, immune, or nervous systems."

---

[21] http://www.who.int/features/qa/87/en/

To play it safe I would buy 100% organic all the time, but I don't for two reasons.

1. It's expensive to buy all organic.

2. Some foods are lower risk than others to humans when it comes to pesticide exposure, so I do my best to avoid the higher risk foods. I sometimes buy non-organic if the foods are lower risk.

Here are two lists from the Environmental Working Group (EWG) to help make your food shopping experience less confusing. These are the lists I use when deciding to buy organic vs. non-organic.

THE DIRTY DOZEN

The first list is known as the Dirty Dozen, which are the 12 foods that the EWG reports have the highest levels of pesticide residue.[22]

The Dirty Dozen	
1. Strawberries	7. Cherries
2. Spinach	8. Grapes
3. Nectarines	9. Celery
4. Apples	10. Tomatoes
5. Peaches	11. Sweet bell peppers
6. Pears	12. Potatoes

---

[22] https://www.ewg.org/foodnews/dirty_dozen_list.php

This list is known as the Clean Fifteen and this is the list with the lowest amount of pesticide residue.[23]

CLEAN FIFTEEN

The Clean Fifteen	
1. Sweet corn	9. Mangos
2. Avocados	10. Eggplant
3. Pineapples	11. Honeydew melon
4. Cabbage	12. Kiwi
5. Onions	13. Cantaloupe
6. Sweet peas, frozen	14. Cauliflower
7. Papayas	15. Grapefruit
8. Asparagus	

I rarely buy organic from the Clean Fifteen unless the price is similar to conventional. Overall, if the extra cost to purchase organic is minimal I will always opt for organic. What is the downside to consuming less potentially harmful toxins?

If you are unsure if a fruit or vegetable is organic, check the sticker for the PLU code:

- If the number starts with a 4, the item is conventional (non-organic). For example, #4011 is the code for a conventional (non-organic) yellow banana.

---

[23] https://www.ewg.org/foodnews/clean_fifteen_list.php

- If the number starts with a 9, the item is organic. For example, #94011 is the code for an organic yellow banana.
- If the number starts with an 8, the item is genetically engineered (GE). For example, #84011 is the code for a genetically engineered yellow banana.

Some experts, like Dr. David Perlmutter, report that there is increasing concern regarding the impact of glyphosate, an ingredient in a popular pesticide. Dr. Perlmutter says that while the science around the issue is still evolving, glyophosate changes the balance of the bacteria in the microbiome,[24] setting the stage for leaky gut and autoimmune disease. What scientists have recently come to understand is that the makeup and health of your microbiome determines whether these bacteria in the gut coexist peacefully, or cause disease.

For those of us who are understandably concerned about the cost to eat healthier, I would encourage you to strongly weigh the risks of not doing so against a small amount of extra investment now.

Few of us need to be reminded of the spiraling costs of health care. As if the rise of our overall premiums are not bad enough, the more recent painful cost for the average American family is the spike in out-of-pocket costs. The average yearly deductible has gone up $486 since 2011.[25] This is before we factor in the rising prescription drug costs, out of network premiums, co-payments, and coinsurance fees! The cost of getting sick in the U.S. is beyond prohibitive at this point and is the *number one cause of bankruptcy.*[26]

---

[24] http://www.drperlmutter.com/pesticides-damage-microbiome/

[25] http://www.businessinsider.com/out-of-pocket-healthcare-payments-skyrocketing-2016-9

[26] https://www.msn.com/en-us/money/personalfinance/this-is-the-no-1-reason-americans-file-for-bankruptcy/ar-BBAAvmY

But these mind-numbing stats do NOT necessarily need to affect us the way they do most people.

The other viable option for most of us to consider is the 'ounce of prevention is worth a pound of cure' vantage point. It is time for us to remember the Father of Medicine, Hippocrates, and his famous words, *"Let food be thy medicine and medicine be thy food."* Hippocrates was referring to the clean, whole foods and not the processed junk that line most of the supermarket aisles!

Simple Step #10: Try to fill your cart with fresh, *whole* foods when you are grocery shopping. Buy organic produce whenever possible, especially if it's found on the Dirty Dozen list. You may be surprised at how affordable and delicious many whole foods can be.

Progress Over Perfection Action Questions:

1. Do you have any digestion issues you are aware of? Are there any particular foods that upset your stomach?

2. Do you suffer from bloating, inflammation, food sensitivities, chronic pain, brain fog/poor memory, depression, and/or fatigue? If so, these conditions have been associated to leaky gut syndrome and you may want to explore (under doctor supervision if necessary) improving your gut's bacteria balance, decreasing your processed food consumption, and increasing your probiotic intake.

3. What is the biggest challenge holding you back from buying whole foods and avoiding processed and fast foods? Is it time, money, and/or convenience? If you knew you could seriously improve your health and reduce your risk of developing chronic illness, would this motivate you to change the way you buy and prepare your food?

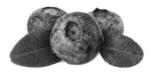

Chapter 6: Calcium, Carbs, and Other Nutritional Shades of Gray

"Any fool can know. The point is to understand."
—Albert Einstein

No other area of science is more fraught with confusion and mixed messages than nutrition. For those of us seeking to improve our wellness journey, this can often feel frustrating and discouraging.

So if this is you, you are not alone.

It certainly doesn't help as we are constantly facing an onslaught of masterfully crafted advertising from the food industry with all kinds of murky claims and promises of nutritional benefits. I cannot emphasize enough the importance of not allowing yourself to get overwhelmed by all the noise out there. One of the simplest remedies to avoiding that feeling of information overload is to focus on consuming a variety of *whole foods* and *do your best to avoid most processed foods (are you noticing a common theme here?)*.

So let's shed some light on some of the grayer areas of nutrition:

Calcium and Vitamin D

Calcium deficiency is the main cause for osteoporosis and low bone mass, currently considered a major public health threat for over 44 million U.S. women and men aged 50 and older.[27] In fact, 50% of women will experience osteoporosis at some point in their life. It is projected that by 2020 more than 61 million women and men will be affected by osteoporosis. With our Standard American Diet (known by the inadvertent yet appropriate acronym—S.A.D.) and current indoor, sedentary lifestyle, our bones are at increasing risk to become weak as we age. It is not uncommon today for the elderly to suffer broken ribs from a sneeze.

So what is a wise preventive measure in order to minimize our risk of osteoporosis and low bone mass? *Consume more calcium!*

Let's take a look at some calcium-rich foods we should aim to include as a part of our daily nutrition.

Foods that are high in calcium:

Spinach	Soybeans	Greek yogurt
Sardines	Kale	Edamame
Salmon	Oatmeal	Oranges

It is ideal to get a balanced intake of most vitamins and minerals through *what we eat.*

Vitamin D in particular is one vitamin known to be *essential* for human health. Sometimes called a steroid vitamin, vitamin D increases the metabolism and the absorption of calcium which helps prevent osteoporosis. In addition, vitamin D promotes cell growth, improves immune function, and reduces inflammation. One of the best sources of vitamin D is exposure to sunlight—of course please keep in mind this needs to be measured against possible skin cancer

---

[27] https://www.iofbonehealth.org/facts-statistics#category-23

risk. Be sure to speak to your dermatologist before spending more time in the sun.

Foods that are high in vitamin D:

Tuna	Sardines	Portobello mushrooms
Egg yolks	Salmon	Sprouted Tofu

Simple Step #11: Get at least 15 minutes of sun exposure every day (but be sure to wear sunscreen and consult your doctor if you are going to be in the sun longer than 15 minutes.) Sunshine is still one of the *best* sources for vitamin D! Even on cloudy days be sure to get outside for those precious minutes.

Salt

As we discussed in Chapter 1, the FDA recommends we limit our daily sodium consumption to 2300 mg—about a teaspoon of salt. Like sugar, salt is drastically overused in our country's food supply, so we should be vigilant in reading our labels and keeping an eye on our intake. In lieu of salt, **try to season foods with herbs and spices such as dill, pepper, turmeric, garlic powder, paprika, cilantro, chives, or curry to name a few.** If you feel you need to salt, it's best to use sea salt over table salt, because it is less processed, although both are believed to have similar nutritional value (or lack of it).

Carbs: Friend or Foe?

The simple fact is that all carbs are NOT bad for us. Good carbohydrates should be a main source of energy in a balanced diet. Many whole foods containing these good carbs are important for us to be consuming daily because they are a key source of fiber, a critically important component to our digestion process. Some examples of these foods which contain the good carbs are:

Vegetables	Whole grains	Legumes (when prepared correctly)
Fruits	Nuts	

The carbs we want to try to avoid are the processed grain-based or sugary carbohydrates. These types of carbs are prevalent in Western diets and most nutritionists agree that they are one of the primary culprits in our nation's obesity epidemic. Overconsumption of these bad carbs leads to fat deposits in the areas of the body where fat is hardest to lose - the hips, butt, and belly. These refined, bad carbs are a prime factor that has led to our nation's current obesity epidemic.

Think about all those snack foods we like to graze on like chips, dips, crackers, and cookies. They offer little to no nutritional value and because of this our bodies won't receive the *"I'm full"* signals. Instead, our bodies are tricked into craving even more in order to reach that feeling of fullness or satiety. At the same time, wild blood sugar swings and insulin surges from an over stimulated pancreas (due to the sugar overload it is forced to deal with all it once) occur and this leads to our incredible, but overworked liver having to step in to shoulder the workload. What does our beleaguered liver do with all this excessive sugar load? It has no choice but to store it as FAT.

So when it comes to carbs let's do our best to *avoid* the following harmful foods loaded with refined carbs:

Cereals	Bagels	Candy	Most supermarket breads
White pasta	Muffins	Sodas	
White rice	Crackers	Fruit Juices	

Overconsumption of these bad carbs leads to fat deposits in the areas of the body where fat is hardest to lose—the hips, butt, and belly.

The Skinny on FAT

Good Fat

Another common nutrition myth is that fat is to blame for our nation's obesity crisis. As we've just learned, bad carbs play an increasingly large role in the rising obesity rates. It is important to understand that not all fats are bad for us. In fact, some types are actually good for us so we want to ensure we are consuming an adequate amount on a daily basis (which is not hard to do). The main types of fats that are good for us are monounsaturated fat and polyunsaturated fats.

Monounsaturated fat comes from a variety of foods and oils. Research has shown that eating foods that contain monounsaturated fat can improve our blood cholesterol level and decrease our risk of cardiovascular disease.

These foods include:

Avocados	Peanut butter	Olive oil
Nuts	Almond butter	

Polyunsaturated fat comes primarily from plant-based foods and oils. Like its good fat sister mono, polyunsaturated fat can decrease our risk of heart disease by lowering blood cholesterol levels. A certain type of this fat you may have heard of, because it gets a lot of attention, is called omega-3 fatty acids, which are particularly beneficial for our heart.

Foods that include polyunsaturated fat are:

Tofu	Walnuts	Sunflower seeds
Salmon	Almond butter	Sunflower oil
Trout	Flaxseed	

Bad Fat

The two types of bad fat are certain sources of saturated fat and trans fat. Both have been identified as contributing to a rise in our total cholesterol levels and may increase our risk of type 2 diabetes. Although some saturated fats are not as harmful as we may have been led to believe, both these types of fat should generally be avoided or in the case of some dairy, enjoyed in occasional moderation. Some examples of foods with saturated fat are:

Cheese	Milk	Ice cream
Butter	Poultry skin	Whipped cream
Fatty Cuts of Beef, Pork, and Lamb		Most fast foods

Trans fat, short for trans-fatty acids, are found in many processed foods that contain partially hydrogenated vegetable oils. These artificial trans fats are the worst types of fat for us and should be avoided whenever possible. Trans fat can raise our LDL or "bad" cholesterol and suppress the levels of our HDL or "good" cholesterol. Artificial trans fats are found in foods such as:

Fried foods	Margarine
Processed snack foods	Packaged baked goods (cookies & cakes)

Simple Step #12: Instead of microwave popcorn that contains harmful artificial trans fat, try popping your own popcorn in a large 3-quart saucepan. Heat 3 tablespoons of coconut or olive oil. Add ½ cup of high quality organic popcorn, cover, and pop until 30 seconds after you hear the last kernel pop. Flavor with olive oil and a little sea salt and you have a delicious healthy treat.

Other Nutritional Shades of Gray

Unfortunately, many mainstream nutritionists, in their quest for fame and fortune, have been spreading dietary myths that have lead to poor health outcomes. These fad diets and bogus dietary theories have only served to confuse the general public and contribute to the "noise" factor that has led many of us astray from a life of health and wellness.

Time to debunk some longstanding myths many of us may still fall prey to. According to the *New York Times* best-selling author Dr. Joseph Mercola, whose website is the most visited natural health website in the world, here are the 10 lies and misconceptions that are spread by mainstream nutrition[28] and refuted by science:

Lie # 1: Saturated Fat Causes Heart Disease

Lie # 2: Eating Fat Makes Us Gain Weight

Lie # 3: Artificial Sweeteners are Safe Sugar-Replacements for Diabetics, and Help Promote Weight Loss

Lie # 4: Your Body Cannot Tell the Difference Between Sugar and Fructose

Lie # 5: Soy is a Health Food

Lie # 6: Eggs are a Source of Unhealthy Cholesterol

Lie # 7: Whole Grains are Good for Everyone

Lie # 8: Milk Does Your Body Good

Lie # 9: Genetically Engineered Foods are Safe and Comparable to Conventional Foods

Lie # 10: Lunch Meats Make for a Healthy Nutritious Meal

Is there universal agreement to these assertions by Dr. Mercola? No.

But where in the world do we find universal agreement? Nowhere. One thing that Dr. Mercola and most other credible nutrition and

---

[28] http://articles.mercola.com/sites/articles/archive/2013/02/25/mainstream-nutrition-biggest-lies.aspx

wellness professionals agree on is that we need to eat clean, whole foods that are AS CLOSE TO NATURE AS POSSIBLE.

Progress Over Perfection Action Questions:

1. Have you felt confused by all the mixed nutritional and dietary messages out there? Is there an area of nutrition where you may have been led astray?
2. What area of nutrition do you find the most confusing and/or frustrating? Have you ever taken a few minutes to research this area?
3. Do you believe that by having a better understanding of food and nutrition you will be more motivated to make healthier choices? Why or why not?

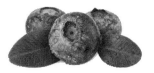

Chapter 7: Moving On Up

"Whether you think you can, or think you can't—you're right."
—Henry Ford

From the time we are born until the time we turn age 30, our muscles grow larger and stronger. At some point in our thirties, we start to lose muscle mass and function. The medical term to describe this physiological reality is sarcopenia. In simple terms, this means, use it or lose it. Physical *inactivity* is not an option if we want to remain healthy. Period.

> Physical *inactivity* is not an option if we want to remain healthy.

Let's consider the choice of having a lifestyle that does not include some physical activity. The experts at WebMD state that "physically *inactive* people can lose as much as 3% to 5% of their muscle mass each decade after age 30."[29] Another term for this condition is (muscle) atrophy. Atrophy is defined by Merriam-Webster dictionary as the gradual loss of muscle or flesh usually because of disease or *lack of use*.[30] The vast majority of cases of atrophy occur as a result of underusing our muscles. This is of particular concern to many health experts today

---

[29] http://www.webmd.com/healthy-aging/sarcopenia-with-aging
[30] https://www.merriam-webster.com/dictionary/atrophy

because of our increasingly sedentary lifestyles. More than ever we are at our desks, in our cars, in front of the TV, or on our smartphones and tablets. For many parents and grandparents of the "just be back home for dinner" generations, it is disturbing to see our helicopter parented children and grandchildren in front of screens for hours each day—at the expense of enjoying the great outdoors. I know because I have been on both sides of this fence. Although I was a kid who was outside running around every chance I got, I have found myself acting like a helicopter parent more times than I would care to admit. Once again, we live in different times and the thought of letting our kids run hog wild as many of us grew up, is perhaps not an option for most parents in this information age of Amber Alerts and perceived sexual predators around every corner.

With our ever-hectic lives, many of us are not carving out the time to MOVE. This is undeniably one of the underlying causes for the massive chronic illness outbreak we have experienced over the past 25 years.

Johns Hopkins Medicine asserts the following health risks associated with physical inactivity[31]:

- Less active and less fit people have a greater risk of developing high blood pressure and are at greater risk for cardiovascular disease.
- Physical activity can reduce your risk for type 2 diabetes
- Studies show that physically active people are less likely to develop coronary heart disease than those who are inactive. This is even after researchers accounted for smoking, alcohol use, and diet.
- Lack of physical activity can add to feelings of anxiety and depression.

---

[31] http://www.hopkinsmedicine.org/healthlibrary/conditions/cardiovascular_diseases/risks_of_physical_inactivity_85,P00218/

- Physical inactivity may increase the risk of certain cancers.
- Physically active overweight or obese people significantly reduced their risk for disease with regular physical activity.

> Physical activity can reduce your risk for type 2 diabetes.

The One Thing We All Agree On!

There is widespread agreement among the medical and wellness community about the benefits of exercise and how much physical activity we need to get. Most experts and institutions like the National Institutes of Health, suggest at least 150 minutes per week of moderate exercise.[32] Ideally, this should include a combination of moderate (walking, cycling) movement to vigorous (jogging, swimming) intense aerobic activity along with strength training (lifting weights, calisthenics). As for structure, 30 minutes of movement, five times per week is considered optimal, so long as we are getting those 150 minutes a week at a minimum of 3 days (50 minutes each) per week we are on the right track. Considering there are 10,080 minutes in a week, 150 min/week (LESS than 1.5% of the total minutes in a week) is really not a lot of time to commit to something so important which we KNOW clearly benefits our overall health. Some of the numerous benefits of incorporating physical activity into your lifestyle are improved cardiovascular health, lower blood pressure, and improved cholesterol levels. It's never too late to get moving!

During a stretch of my own life before my mindful wellness journey began, I was barely working out at all. At my annual

---

[32] https://www.nhlbi.nih.gov/health/health-topics/topics/phys/recommend

physical, my doctor informed me that my overall cholesterol was 240 (200 is the acceptable upper limit). With a history of high cholesterol in my family, and not wanting to go down the prescription path, I began exercising regularly again. The next time I saw my doctor, less than one year later, my cholesterol was down to 192.

Considering there are 10,080 minutes in a week, 150 min/week is really not a lot of time to commit to something so important which we KNOW clearly benefits our overall health. You can do it!.

Being Active Is Good For Your Wallet

A recent study done on more than 26,000 people that was published by the *Journal of the American Heart Association* found that walking just 30 minutes, five days a week can *save us over $3,000 a year* in medical costs.[33] The savings were calculated by looking at the primary cardiovascular related healthcare expenditures which include outpatient visits, hospitalizations, and prescription medications. Besides the cost savings from less doctor visits, we could easily surmise the need for less medical care was due to the study participants FEELING BETTER. You mean I can save money and feel better at the same time? Yep!

What is the risk for *not* staying physically active? Perhaps a higher risk of death or a greater chance of developing a chronic illness, along with less disposable income from the likely added medical costs.

What are we waiting for? Lace up those sneakers and let's get moving.

---

[33] http://jaha.ahajournals.org/content/5/9/e003614

If scheduling the time for physical activity in your busy life seems intimidating at first, you are not alone. Many of us, including myself have been there. Remember, exercise does not have to be in a gym. There are many different options. The important factor is that you find something you enjoy (or at least not consider drudgery) and begin to make it part of your routine.

There is also often a social benefit from exercising. As a result of our over-booked schedules and dependence on technology, many of us are leading more isolated lives today. Exercising is a great way to find a work out buddy; reconnect with a spouse, partner, or friend; or come together as a family.

Simple Step #13: Choose physical activities you like and which are practical. If you don't know whether you will like something, be open-minded and at least give it a try.

Here are a few different physical activities for you to consider doing:

- Swimming
- Running/wind sprints
- Walking (brisk)
- Dance classes
- Cycling/spinning
- Boxing workout
- Cables such as TRX system (very easy to use virtually anywhere you have a door that locks)
- Simple calisthenics like push-ups, sit-ups, and pull-ups—tried, true, and still effective
- Kettlebells

- Yoga
- Pilates
- Tennis/Racquetball
- Volleyball
- Basketball
- Jumping rope
- Soccer
- X-Country skiing
- Numerous home-based workouts found on YouTube
- Gym and studio classes to accommodate everyone's personal taste

Progress Over Perfection Action Questions:

1. What role does physical activity play in your life? Do you get at least the recommended minimum of 150 minutes per week?

2. If regular physical activity is not a part of your life, what do you think is preventing you from doing so? Work, kids, or lack of time? If you are a parent and feel guilty about time away from family, remember the airplane oxygen mask rule—put on your own oxygen mask before helping those around you. A healthier YOU makes you a better caretaker!

3. Who can support you in getting started? Have you ever tried asking a friend, colleague, or loved one to join you?

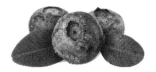

Chapter 8: Ree-Lax

"Nothing can bring you peace but yourself."
—Ralph Waldo Emerson

Relax. Chill out. Slow down. Take it easy.

As we all know, this is easier said than done—especially in today's over connected world. So many of my clients are extremely stressed out—feeling like the proverbial hamster on the wheel. Managing the balancing act of career, family, friends, and finances is more stressful than ever in this 100 mph world. Today, the stresses of modern life permeate every corner of our society and their effect on our physical and psychological wellbeing should not be underestimated.

୬

Stress

There are two types of stress. One (eustress) is good and the other (distress) is not.

The good kind (eustress) is the stress that comes from our natural hardwiring for survival as a means of protection when faced with an emergency situation—a burning house or a negative bank balance when our rent or mortgage is due. Most often, when we experience this type of stress it compels us to complete a given task or goal. For example, preparing to host a holiday party or getting our taxes done before the deadline are examples of this good type of stress. The bad kind is the type of stress that occurs daily over a longer duration, such as being in a toxic relationship, severe financial hardship, or having a boss with unreasonable expectations. This bad type of stress can become chronic over time and cause serious damage to our health as well as our ability to function optimally.

According to researchers at the Mayo Clinic, the long-term activation of the stress-response system, and the subsequent overexposure to cortisol and other stress hormones, can disrupt almost all of our body's processes[34].

This puts us at increased risk for numerous health problems, including:

- Anxiety
- Depression
- Digestive problems
- Headaches
- Heart disease
- Sleep problems
- Weight gain
- Memory and concentration impairment

Our focus needs to be on reducing or eliminating this harmful type of chronic stress from our lives.

In order to attain a higher degree of relaxation and stress relief in our lives we need to be very intentional in how we approach a solution. In other words we need to make its attainment a real priority. Healthy, sustainable relaxation does not happen accidently.

---

[34] http://www.mayoclinic.org/healthy-lifestyle/stress-management/in-depth/stress/art-20046037

> In order to attain a higher degree of relaxation and stress *relief* in our lives we need to be very intentional in how we approach a solution. Healthy, sustainable relaxation does not happen accidently.

Despair Gives Courage to the Coward

At one point, stress was literally sucking the life out of me. I had three children, struggling businesses in NYC, Miami, and South America, a crumbling marriage, and the stranglehold of the Great Recession, which was rapidly turning profitable ventures unprofitable. Eventually in 2009 a challenging divorce entered the mix and with three young children who needed me more than ever, my stress level reached a fever pitch.

As someone who took great pride in being able to come up with a solution for any challenge, I was unable to do so this time. I was out of answers and despite being blessed with some occasional support from friends and family, it was clear major change needed to happen.

But before I went to that wonderful place of surrender, change, and exploration, I needed my world to be rocked even more.

ℰᴑ

In 2007, my business career had peaked. I had just finished the first year of a program at an Ivy League business school where I spent three weeks living with international movers and shakers. On the last day of school I had closed on the purchase of a piece of commercial real estate on one of Manhattan's premier blocks. My first order of business after sealing the deal? Joining the prestigious Harvard Club which happened to be across the street from our new real estate acquisition. Walking down West 44th Street, I remember feeling like I had the world on a string. The "power and money world" of Manhattan can be intoxicating.

Less than 24 hours later, my world seemed to be falling apart. After a series of events within a short 90-minute timeframe, it became abundantly clear to me that my already faltering marriage was in complete shambles. I was devastated by what appeared to be an irreparable situation. In despair, I began frantically pacing back and forth trying to sort everything out in my head. There had to be an escape hatch to this nightmare.

My normally optimistic brain was unable to come up with a solution. I remember thinking of my three young children and how a divorce might affect them. The pain was stinging; my heart was racing out of my chest, and I felt like I was in the chokehold of a panic attack.

A bit of momentary solace was found when I reached a friend on the phone who was able to calm me down a bit. Over the next three weeks I could not sleep and barely ate a morsel of food. Fun times.

As Thomas Fuller, the 17th-century English writer once said, "Despair gives courage to the coward."

ဢ

There was a huge silver lining for me from this experience.

I had finally reached the point where I realized I needed to change from the inside out, and not the outside in. Reaching out for help and being open to the wisdom I was receiving allowed me to explore and grow as a person in ways I had never fully understood. I began with counseling, Al-Anon (a support group for friends and families of problem drinkers), yoga, meditation, and exploring faith. It hasn't always been easy, but the journey of self-exploration has been rewarding beyond measure. I acquired, and am still acquiring, tools that I have found invaluable for navigating my life.

The lesson I learned and like to share from my personal journey is that we do NOT need to wait for tragedy to strike in order to pursue positive change within ourselves. I learned and choose to live by the belief that I am a work in progress. We get one shot at this life, so stagnation is not an option for me.

It's important to note that self-improvement requires a balanced approach just like our approach to overall wellness. Pursuing self-growth that is solely or overly rooted in self-gratification or self-glorification is not necessarily healthy either. Many of us have watched someone we know radically transform their body by going to the gym and then become obsessed with their "new" body—leading to excessive time spent in the gym at the expense of other areas of their life.

In my own case I discovered I needed to improve my patience, parenting skills, and ability to be more compassionate. Most of my heightened awareness and growth came from meditation, conscious listening, and prayer. Sometimes doing nothing, being still, present, and allowing ourselves to listen is the best form of relaxation and mindfulness.

Seeking conscious relaxation and understanding how to reduce the stress in our lives, like any other goal, begins with that first step.

Breathe with Me

Dr. Andrew Weil, the well-known Harvard Medical School trained doctor and founder of the Arizona Center for Integrative Medicine recommends a very simple, yet effective breathing practice known as the 4-7-8 Breath (a.k.a. the Relaxing Breath) which "puts the practitioner in a relaxed state almost immediately." It takes a couple minutes, requires no equipment, and can be done anywhere. Let's give it a try!

Although you can do the exercise in any position, it helps if you start by sitting with your back straight. Place the tip of your tongue against the ridge of tissue just behind your upper front teeth, and keep it there through the entire exercise. You will be exhaling through your mouth around your tongue; try pursing your lips slightly if this seems awkward.

1. Exhale completely through your mouth, making a whoosh sound.
2. Close your mouth and inhale quietly through your nose to a mental count of **4**.
3. Hold your breath for a count of **7**.
4. Exhale completely through your mouth, making a whoosh sound to a count of **8**.
5. This is one breath. Now inhale again and repeat the cycle three more times for a total of four breaths.

> Sometimes doing nothing, being still, present, and allowing ourselves to listen is the best form of relaxation and mindful growth.

I regularly practice the 4-7-8 breathing technique and it always brings me a sense of relaxation and calmness. What's important to remember is that the pursuit of relaxation is far more than a temporary reprieve from our daily stress. It may begin as such, but with consistent practice these stress reduction activities can lead to tremendous gain—physically, emotionally, and spiritually.

Mindfulness—the gateway to experiencing our optimal wellness

For those of us who wish to also try (and I strongly encourage this) another form of relaxation, there is the very simple yet powerfully effective practice of meditation.

Because of its Eastern roots, there are many false perceptions about meditation. It is important to know that meditation does NOT need to be associated with any organized religion. There are numerous forms of meditation that have nothing to do with Buddha or any other higher power. You can easily find types of meditation that are Christian or Jewish or secularly-based. Most of the web-based apps you will find out there do not have any religious undertones. What matters the most, is that you choose a style that feels most comfortable for YOU.

The comedian Jerry Seinfeld is a well-known practitioner of Transcendental Meditation (TM). He is outspoken about the invaluable benefits he has experienced from his daily commitment. In fact, he attributes much of his professional and personal success to his daily practice of 20 minutes of meditation. While doing the TV show that bore his name, he famously wore many hats—actor, executive producer, writer, editor, and casting director—each a full time stressful job in their own right requiring serious accountability and responsibility. He openly shares that there is no way he could have survived that grueling schedule for nine years without his daily meditation practice. It's no surprise that at age 62 he looks younger than many 40-year-olds. Although Seinfeld's career is not run of the mill, the enormous benefits he derived from meditation are par for the course. Like the wonderful benefits we enjoy from eating more raw leafy green vegetables—this stuff works.

Why does it work? There are many reasons for its efficacy, but the essence of meditation's success centers around the change in brain activity. From the simple act of mindful breathing (which is at the heart of nearly all forms of meditation), we place our bodies in a state of stillness and relaxation. Over time this state allows for an increase in gray matter concentration in key areas of our brain. Gray matter is the neural tissue of the brain and spinal cord that contains nerve cell bodies and nerve fibers. Increasing gray matter concentration in our brain has been associated with improved memory, learning, and emotion.[35]

Sara Lazar, PhD, led a study at Harvard in 2011 that found meditation increased cortical thickness in the hippocampus, the part of the brain that governs learning and memory. She and her team of researchers found evidence that "meditation may slow down the age related atrophy of certain areas of the brain."[36] Who wouldn't want to expand the area of our brain that can lead to improved memory without having to undergo any surgery at no cost?

> Sara Lazar, PhD, led a study at Harvard in 2011 that found meditation increased cortical thickness in the hippocampus, the part of the brain that governs learning and memory.

Dr. Herbert Benson, the best selling author of *The Relaxation Response*, is known as one of the modern Western experts on meditation as well as the harmful effects of stress. He has been quoted as saying, "Modern science has shown us that the mind has the power to heal. We should use that capacity." Dr. Benson founded the Benson-Henry Institute for Mind Body Medicine at the

---

[35] https://nccih.nih.gov/research/results/spotlight/012311.htm
[36] https://scholar.harvard.edu/sara_lazar/home

Massachusetts General Hospital which works to integrate modern scientific medicine, psychology, nutrition, exercise physiology, and faith, with the expectation that this will enhance the natural healing capacities of body and mind. His research indicates that practicing the relaxation response (e.g., meditation) produces immediate changes in the expression of genes involved in immune function, energy metabolism, and insulin secretion. In the film documentary *The Connection: Mind Your Body*, a number of patients were filmed who were adding Dr. Benson's mind-body programs to their chronic illness treatment strategy. It was found that diabetes, hypertension, heart disease, autoimmune disease, fatigue, and stress-induced conditions like chronic headaches are all illnesses responding well to his programs.

> The importance of having a MINDFULNESS practice in our lives is science based. "Modern science has shown us that the mind has the power to heal. We should use that capacity."
> —Dr. Herbert Benson

The benefits for us do not end there. In a controlled clinical study at the University of Wisconsin it was found that "meditation may change immune function in positive ways."[37] So add the possibility of boosting our immune systems to the other invaluable attributes of practicing meditation!

The success of practicing meditation and other forms of mindfulness is now so widespread it has been implemented in public schools, hospitals, and even prisons. At the Robert W. Coleman Elementary School in Baltimore, there are approximately 300 students who participate in the "Mindful Moments" program,

---

[37] https://www.sciencedaily.com/releases/2003/02/030204074125.htm

learning to breathe, stretch, and block out distractions, while doing a 15 minute blend of yoga and meditation every morning. Additionally, instead of using a traditional detention setting or the principal's office as a disciplinary approach, the youthful offenders are sent to the Mindful Me Room, an oasis of colorful tapestries with beanbag chairs, oil diffusers, and herbal tea, where they practice deep-breathing exercises, meditate, and talk about what happened when conflict arises.[38] Students are taught to redirect negative energy into something positive. Since initiating the program, *there have been zero suspensions.* And this is in Baltimore, where there is a prevalence of crime and drug abuse in many of the city's neighborhoods.

> The success of practicing meditation and other forms of mindfulness is so widespread it has been implemented in public schools, hospitals, and even prisons.

Although I was aware of the incredible benefits people experienced from practicing meditation and other relaxation techniques like deep breathing or prayer, I put off doing it for a long time. I had a laundry list of excuses—too busy, don't know how, won't be able to sit still for that long, but truthfully, I was intimidated by what I did not fully understand and had absolutely no experience doing. When I finally decided to take the plunge and began to meditate I discovered two things—it was SO easy to learn and I immediately experienced the incredible benefits I had heard so much about.

Like anything else, don't knock it until you try it!

---

[38] https://www.sciencedaily.com/releases/2003/02/030204074125.htm

Simple Step #14: Do a Google or YouTube search for *free meditation* or *relaxation techniques*. This is a simple, easy way to begin your journey to reduce stress in your life and incorporate a mindfulness practice. Take five minutes and start today. There are also a number of free apps you can check out. I recommend downloading Insight Timer, Aura, or Headspace. You can track your progress and become part of a global meditation community

Progress Over Perfection Action Questions:

1. How does stress show up in your life? How does it affect you?

2. How does stress impact your relationships with family? Coworkers? Friends?

3. What do you think it would feel like if you had less stress in your life?

4. Have you often felt like that hamster on the wheel? Do you currently have any kind of mindfulness practice in your life? It could be as simple as a walk, quiet reflective time, prayer...etc.

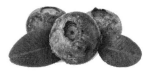

Chapter 9: Snooze It or Lose It

*"And he said to them, 'Come away by yourselves
to a desolate place and rest a while.'"*
—The Bible, Mark 6:31

Getting adequate sleep is vital in order to maintain our ideal health and wellness.

Despite the massive amounts of credible evidence proving this to be the case, this was the one area of my overall health that I stubbornly resisted accepting as the truism that it is. My mother used to tell me years ago about the importance of sleep yet I would unwisely counter that life is too short to sleep or that I was fine as long as I got five hours a night. During this time I was an entrepreneur, living and working in New York City, and subscribing to the false notion that sleep was for wimps. Boy, was I wrong! Besides the overall detrimental effect on my body and mind from not getting enough sleep, I had two near-death experiences from falling asleep at the wheel of a car before the age of 30.

According to the National Institutes of Health (NIH), "Sleep plays a vital role in good health and wellbeing throughout your life. Getting enough quality sleep at the right times can help protect your mental health, physical health, quality of life, and safety."[39]

For example, sleep is involved in the healing and repair of our

---

[39] https://www.nhlbi.nih.gov/health/health-topics/topics/sdd/why

hearts and blood vessels. Ongoing sleep deficiency is linked to an increased risk of heart disease, kidney disease, high blood pressure, diabetes, and stroke. Multiple studies have also shown that sleep deprived individuals gain more weight than their well-rested counterparts. So add increased risk of being overweight and obesity to the list of risks associated with not getting sufficient sleep.

Multiple studies have also shown that sleep deprived individuals gain more weight than their well-rested counterparts.

The graph below, from a study conducted by the National Health and Nutrition Examination Survey (NHANES) over a three-year period, revealed the following differences in people performing activities based on sleep duration. In virtually every activity area, the participants getting less than seven hours of sleep per night performed *less well* than those who reported getting more than seven hours.[40]

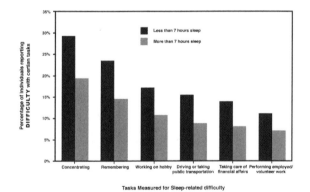

[40] https://www.cdc.gov/mmwr/preview/mmwrhtml/mm6008a3.htm

Scientists from the University of Wisconsin recently discovered that *sleep increases the reproduction of cells* that form myelin. Myelin is the insulating material found on nerve cell projections in the brain and spinal cord that are responsible for allowing electrical impulses to move from cell to cell, similar to insulation around an electrical wire.[41] Just like an electrical wire needs insulation to protect the electrical currents, our bodies need myelin to protect the nerve impulses that carry messages from one part of our body to another. Our bodies are comprised of literally trillions of these important cells which are protected by myelin. *Sleep is crucial to enabling these cells to perform optimally and regenerate.*

> Sleep is involved in the healing and repair of our hearts and blood vessels.

Sleep Your Way to the Top

In Arianna Huffington's recent book *The Sleep Revolution*, she candidly addresses what she refers to as "Our Current Sleep Crisis".[42] She points out the irony of society's view around sleep and productivity— "In the name of productivity we forego sleep, but in fact our productivity is actually *reduced substantially* when we're sleep deprived." Huffington is passionate about the subject because the data proves the detrimental consequences to "every aspect of our health" including some that should give us all pause—hypertension (less snooze means a harder time processing stress, leading to higher blood pressure), a suppressed immune system (may be why some of

---

[41] http://www.medicalnewstoday.com/articles/265678.php
[42] http://www.ariannahuffington.com/books/the-sleep-revolution-hc

us are always getting that cold), and obesity (the sleepy folks crave bad carbs and sugars). She wittily encourages youth to "sleep their way to the top." OK, sounds great, but what if I have a hard time falling asleep or continually wake up during the night and can't fall *back* to sleep?

"In the name of productivity we forego sleep, but in fact our productivity is actually *reduced substantially* when we're sleep deprived."

Here's a list of nine ways to help you get a good night's sleep:

1. Exercise—Movement is proven to enhance the sleep quality in adults. Yoga might top the list for most effective exercises here, but remember to aim for those 150 minutes per week of physical activity which ideally includes both cardio and strength training.

2. Meditate—Several studies show that regular meditation practice results in higher blood levels of melatonin[43] (which decreases the amount of time it takes us to fall asleep), an important regulator of sleep.[44]

3. Cut down on sugar intake, especially in the evening. Of the numerous bad effects of excessive sugar consumption, interfering with our sleep is one caused by a spike in our blood sugar that makes it harder to stay and fall asleep.

---

[43] https://www.brainwave-research-institute.com/how-meditation-boosts-melatonin-production.html
[44] http://www.webmd.com/sleep-disorders/alternative_treatments_for_insomnia#2

4. Lose weight—many studies have shown that people who are significantly overweight or obese are likely to report insomnia or difficulty with sleep.

5. Avoid drinking any liquids past 8 p.m. to reduce nighttime trips to the bathroom.

6. Include lots of dark leafy greens in your diet.

7. Regularly drink *organic* green and chamomile teas—both contain compounds proven to enhance sleep quality. Although green tea does contain caffeine, so you may want to avoid at night, it also contains the amino acid L-theanine, which can enhance the quality of our sleep.[45]

8. Eat some almonds after dinner. Almonds contain magnesium, which promotes both sleep and muscle relaxation.

9. Put away or turn off all electronic devices when getting ready for bedtime. The light emanating from our devices can often trick our bodies into thinking it's daytime.

According to Dr. Judith Owens, the director of the Center for Pediatric Sleep Disorders at Boston Children's Hospital, getting enough sleep is "just as important as good nutrition, physical activity, and wearing your seat belt."[46] With two-thirds of Americans not getting enough sleep, according to a National Sleep Foundation report, ensuring healthy sleep habits is something that we need to start taking much more seriously.

---

[45] http://www.nutraingredients.com/Research/Green-tea-lulls-brain-into-quality-sleep
[46] http://ariannahuffington.com/books/the-sleep-revolution-tr/the-sleep-revolution-hc

> Getting enough sleep is "just as important as good nutrition, physical activity, and wearing your seat belt."

Proper sleep habits are so important to our overall wellbeing that there is even said to be a proven link between effective leadership and getting enough sleep. Nick van Dam, a McKinsey & Co. principal and visiting professor at Harvard and the University of Pennsylvania, writes in the *Harvard Business Review*[47] that one of the areas of the brain most responsible for effective executive functioning is the prefrontal cortex which controls our cognitive processes such as problem solving, reasoning, organization, and executive functioning. He points out that neuroscientists know that although some areas of the brain can cope relatively well with too little sleep, the prefrontal cortex cannot. It is more obvious that sleep deprivation very often causes deterioration of basic visual and motor skills (that groggy feeling we get when we are overtired and do something like put the box of cereal in the fridge). To most of us it is less obvious that the area of the brain most associated with our executive functioning and organizational skills is actually impaired when we don't get enough sleep.[48] Now that we know about the possible consequences to our brain, let's ensure our prefrontal cortex is not being deprived by aiming to get more shut-eye!

Another solution to experiment with is as simple as sticking to consistent times for your sleep. As reported by *BBC News*, independent sleep consultant Dr. Neil Stanley is quoted saying, "The most effective way to improve your sleep is to fix your wake-

---

[47] https://hbr.org/2016/02/theres-a-proven-link-between-effective-leadership-and-getting-enough-sleep

[48] https://sleepfoundation.org/media-center/press-release/annual-sleep-america-poll-exploring-connections-communications-technology-use-

up time in the morning. Your body craves regularity, so if you chop and change your sleep pattern, your body hasn't got a clue when it should prepare to wake up or not."[49] Try getting into the habit of going to bed and waking up at the same time every day.

Despite the challenges for some, sleep is still considered one of the easiest of the health and wellbeing pillars. Many cherish the act. Who doesn't enjoy rest when they are tired?

> **Simple Step #15:** Do yourself a big favor and make sleep a priority! As an adult, aim to get at *least* seven hours of sleep each night.

---

[49] http://www.bbc.com/future/story/20150706-the-woman-who-barely-sleeps

Progress Over Perfection Action Questions:

1. How many hours of sleep do you average a night? If you are getting less than seven, what is the reason?

2. Do you ever feel like you can't afford to get more sleep or worry that if you did, something important in your life would have to be sacrificed?

3. What would have to change in your life for you to be able to get a minimum of seven hours of sleep per night? Are you truly committed to urgent matters 17 hours a day or are there certain habits such as watching TV or trolling social media that could be cut down a bit?

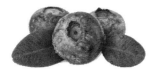

Chapter 10: Giving = Living

"No act of kindness, no matter how small, is ever wasted."

—Aesop

A struggling young waitress in LA was about to have her best shift ever.

Chelsea's life hadn't been easy. She raised her little sister from a young age and overcame an eating disorder. Despite her challenges, she always went out of her way to help others. Recognizing her tireless good attitude and generous spirit, her boss and colleagues at the restaurant arranged a series of pleasant surprises.

Chelsea's first customer came in and left her a $1,000 cash tip, which she immediately wanted to share with her coworkers. Soon after, a couple explained that they had just enough to pay the tab although no cash for a tip, BUT were travel agents and happened to have two free plane tickets to Hawaii they wanted to give her. Next, a woman offered Chelsea her dream job as a yoga instructor. Her last customer placed in the bill holder a key to a brand new car that was parked outside the restaurant—complete with a big red bow! And finally a dear friend from her past was flown in as part of the surprise waiting to meet her in front of her brand new car as she was led outside the restaurant.[50]

Who is the real beneficiary here? Chelsea?

---

[50] https://www.youtube.com/watch?v=p2zUf06iy1A&feature=youtu.be

Guess again. It is the givers NOT the recipients who actually benefit the most. In this case, the beneficiaries are her boss and coworkers who arranged the day and gave of themselves so Chelsea could receive that altruistic bounty.

You *Can* Buy Happiness

According to researchers at Harvard, *you can actually buy happiness*—but ONLY if you give it away. Even giving "as little as $5 can lead to increased wellbeing for the giver." The joint study by one Harvard and two University of British Columbia professors found that "it was the relative percentage of their money that people spent on others—rather than the absolute amount that predicted their happiness."[51]

Of course the benefits of giving are not restricted to monetary gifts. Giving of our time, our talents, and just being compassionate with those around us have a direct positive impact on our health. In his book *The Compassionate Achiever*, author Christopher Kukk, PhD, writes that "when we think compassionately, we use the same neural pathways as love. Because compassion is connected to love, we are nourished."[52]

So where's the link between love and better health? An article from Medicinenet.com entitled *10 Surprising Health Benefits of Love* lists the research-backed ways that health and love are connected[53]:

---

[51] http://hbswk.hbs.edu/item/spending-on-happiness
[52] The Compassionate Achiever (book), page 2. Author: Christopher L Kukk, Phd
[53] http://www.medicinenet.com/script/main/art.asp?articlekey=97679

1. Fewer Doctor Visits
2. Less Depression and Substance Abuse
3. Lower Blood Pressure
4. Less Anxiety
5. Natural Pain Control
6. Better Stress Management
7. Fewer Colds
8. Faster Healing
9. Longer Life
10. Happier Life

> When we think compassionately, we use the same neural pathways as love. Because compassion is connected to love, we are nourished.

We all have unique forms of expression for showing and desiring love as evidenced in the *New York Times* best selling book, *The Five Love Languages* by Dr. Gary Chapman. Dr. Chapman teaches that we express and receive love through one of five languages: words of affirmation, quality time, receiving gifts, acts of service, or physical touch. He states that "while each one of these languages is enjoyed to some degree by all people, a person will usually speak one primary language."[54]

Giving is good for our health

There is a wide range of research that has linked different forms of generosity to better health, even among the sick and elderly. Stephen Post, PhD, a professor at Stony Brook University, and

---

[54] https://en.wikipedia.org/wiki/Gary_Chapman

author of the book *Why Good Things Happen to Good People,* reports that giving to others has been shown to increase the health benefits in people with chronic illness.[55]

One reason for this boost to our health is related to the positive effect giving has on our stress levels. One joint study by Rachel Piferi of Johns Hopkins University and Kathleen Lawler of the University of Tennessee suggest that one reason giving may improve physical health and longevity is that it helps decrease stress, which is associated with a variety of health problems as we learned. The study indicated that people who provided social support to others had lower blood pressure than participants who didn't, suggesting a direct physiological benefit to those who give of themselves.[56]

Simple Step #16: Make a concerted effort to perform at least one act of giving every week, regardless of how small a gesture. Over time, try to increase your giving frequency to once per day.

Here is a short list of some possible acts of giving to help get you started:

1. Bring a colleague a cup of tea or coffee
2. Donate to a local charity
3. Offer to babysit for a friend or family member who may not be able to afford a sitter
4. Visit elderly members in your community at an assisted living facility

---

[55] https://greatergood.berkeley.edu/article/item/5_ways_giving_is_good_for_you/
[56] https://greatergood.berkeley.edu/article/item/5_ways_giving_is_good_for_you/

5. Surprise someone with a small gift such as a book or a gift card to their favorite lunch spot

6. Offer to help out with someone's pet(s)

7. Pay for a stranger's tab at a restaurant

8. Mentor an at-risk-youth

9. Donate a used book to a library

10. Send someone a hand-written card to let them know you're thinking of them

Our body, mind, and spirit are all nourished when we perform a simple act of kindness. Make it a habit and keep in mind it is important to give without any expectations of receiving anything back. It is also contagious, so get ready to experience its amazing ripple effect!

> Our body, mind, and spirit are all nourished when we perform a simple act of kindness.

Progress Over Perfection Action Questions:

1. When was the last time you performed a simple act of giving? How did it make you feel?

2. If you haven't performed a random act of kindness recently, what might be holding you back from doing so?

3. What are a few simple acts of giving that you could see yourself doing this week?

Conclusion

"Always remember that your future is determined
by what you do today, not tomorrow."
—Robert T. Kiyosaki

Think about those choices we've made that have impacted our lives:

- Reluctantly accepting that invitation to the wedding where you end up meeting your future spouse
- Choosing to speak to that stranger on the plane who ended up offering you a job
- Accepting an invite to join a friend at their church or place of worship which led to a walk of faith

Seemingly insignificant choices can have an enormous impact on our lives.

ॐ

My choosing to embrace a life of health and wellness eight years ago was one of those choices. I no longer live in fear of getting sick. I have more energy, more quality time with my family, virtually no medical expenses, and more zest for life. It was not always this way.

The Butterfly Effect

The Butterfly Effect is a concept suggesting that small causes may have momentous effects. The inventor of the concept, meteorologist Edward N. Lorenz, famously illustrated the concept with the metaphorical question, "Does the flap of a butterfly's wings in Brazil set a tornado in Texas?"[57]

The fact of the matter is that *even the smallest choices* we make can and do have enormous consequences. My invitation to you is to begin to make small changes that could very well lead to a positively changed life for you and your loved ones.

໑

Begin to embrace the evidence-backed concept of "lifestyle as medicine" and explore taking more responsibility for your own health. David L. Katz, MD, MPH, the Yale-trained founder of The True Health Initiative poignantly sums up the dilemma we face:

"As a preventive medicine specialist and current president of the American College of Lifestyle Medicine, the second most frustrating thing in my world is how little we do with what we know. We know how to prevent fully 80 percent of all chronic disease and premature death in the United States, and in industrialized countries around the world. We know how to add years to life and life to years. The failure to do it is the *second* most frustrating thing in my world."

He goes on to say: "I trust this begs the obvious question. What on earth could possibly be the first most frustrating thing? *"Quite simply, knowing that we are paying for the second with the literal lives of our children and our grandchildren."*

We cannot get yesterday back, but you can begin your journey to greater wellness today. Know that our time together does not conclude with this book.

[57] http://www.scholarpedia.org/article/Butterfly_effect#Butterfly_effect.2C_causality_and_chance

I invite you to visit my website www.GreggCRoberts.com to become part of my community. There's a free gift waiting for you that was designed to keep you focused on your health and wellness goals.

Remember: *Progress Over Perfection* along with some Simple Wisdom is THE key to long-term wellbeing success.

It's your move! I know you can do this.

References

We have compiled all references from each chapter of the book for your convenience. For easier access to an online version of these references please visit: www.greggcroberts.com/book-references

Introduction

[1] http://www.npr.org/sections/health-shots/2016/12/08/504667607/life-expectancy-in-u-s-drops-for-first-time-in-decades-report-finds

Chapter 1 – The Problem

[2] https://www.cdc.gov/nchs/data/databriefs/db219.pdf

[3] http://www.unitedhealthgroup.com/newsroom/articles/news/united health%20group/2010/1123whitepaper5usdiabetes.aspx

[4] http://www.cnn.com/2014/02/04/health/who-world-cancer-report/index.html

[5 & 6] https://sodiumbreakup.heart.org/how_much_sodium_should_i_eat

Chapter 2 – Rocket Fuel

[7] https://www.karger.com/Article/Pdf/339375

[8] http://www.medscape.com/viewarticle/717030

[9] http://www.Gerson.org

[10] https://www.sciencedaily.com/releases/2008/04/080430204519.htm

[11] http://www.webmd.com/food-recipes/features/health-benefits-of-green-tea#1

[12] https://www.niaaa.nih.gov/alcohol-health/overview-alcohol-consumption/moderate-binge-drinking

Chapter 3 – What We See Is Not What We Get

[13] http://www.heart.org/HEARTORG/healthyliving/healthyeating/Nutrition/Sugar-101_UCM_306024_Article.jsp#.wvuotiwcfae

[14] http://www.newyorker.com/magazine/2014/11/03/grain

[15] http://naturallysavvy.com/eat/scary-ingredients-used-in-bread-manufacturing

[16] http://www.newyorker.com/magazine/2014/11/03/grain

[17] http://www.motherjones.com/food/2013/12/cow-feed-chicken-poop-candy-sawdust/

Chapter 5 – Gut Outta Here

[18] https://cspinet.org/resource/food-dyes-rainbow-risks

[19] http://healthpsych.psy.vanderbilt.edu/healthpsych/msg.htm

[20] http://www.livestrong.com/article/345172-the-best-non-fattening-snack-foods/

[21] http://www.who.int/features/qa/87/en/

[22] https://www.ewg.org/foodnews/dirty_dozen_list.php

[23] https://www.ewg.org/foodnews/clean_fifteen_list.php

[24] http://www.drperlmutter.com/pesticides-damage-microbiome/

[25] http://www.businessinsider.com/out-of-pocket-healthcare-payments-skyrocketing-2016-9

[26] https://www.msn.com/en-us/money/personalfinance/this-is-the-no-1-reason-americans-file-for-bankruptcy/ar-bbaavmy

Chapter 6 – Calcium, Carbs, and Other Nutritional Shades of Gray

[27] https://www.iofbonehealth.org/facts-statistics#category-23

[28] http://articles.mercola.com/sites/articles/archive/2013/02/25/mainstream-nutrition-biggest-lies.aspx

Chapter 7 – Moving on Up

[29] http://www.webmd.com/healthy-aging/sarcopenia-with-aging

[30] https://www.merriam-webster.com/dictionary/atrophy

[31] http://www.hopkinsmedicine.org/healthlibrary/conditions/cardiovascular_diseases/risks_of_physical_inactivity_85,P00218/

[32] https://www.nhlbi.nih.gov/health/health-topics/topics/phys/recommend

[33] http://jaha.ahajournals.org/content/5/9/e003614

Chapter 8 – Ree-Lax

[34] http://www.mayoclinic.org/healthy-lifestyle/stress-management/in-depth/stress/art-20046037

[35] https://nccih.nih.gov/research/results/spotlight/012311.htm

[36] https://scholar.harvard.edu/sara_lazar/home

[37 & 38] https://www.sciencedaily.com/releases/2003/02/030204074125.htm

Chapter 9 – Snooze It or Lose It

[39] https://www.nhlbi.nih.gov/health/health-topics/topics/sdd/why

[40] https://www.cdc.gov/mmwr/preview/mmwrhtml/mm6008a3.htm

[41] http://www.medicalnewstoday.com/articles/265678.php

[42] http://www.ariannahuffington.com/books/the-sleep-revolution-hc

[43] https://www.brainwave-research-institute.com/how-meditation-boosts-melatonin-production.html

[44] http://www.webmd.com/sleep-disorders/alternative_treatments_for_insomnia#2

[45] http://www.nutraingredients.com/Research/Green-tea-lulls-brain-into-quality-sleep

[46] http://ariannahuffington.com/books/the-sleep-revolution-tr/the-sleep-revolution-hc

[47] https://hbr.org/2016/02/theres-a-proven-link-between-effective-leadership-and-getting-enough-sleep

[48] https://sleepfoundation.org/media-center/press-release/annual-sleep-america-poll-exploring-connections-communications-technology-use-

[49] http://www.bbc.com/future/story/20150706-the-woman-who-barely-sleeps

Chapter 10 – Giving = Living

[50] https://www.youtube.com/watch?V=p2zuf06iy1a&feature=youtu.be

[51] http://hbswk.hbs.edu/item/spending-on-happiness

[52] The Compassionate Achiever (book), page 2. Author: Christopher L Kukk, Phd

[53] http://www.medicinenet.com/script/main/art.asp?Articlekey=97679

[54] https://en.wikipedia.org/wiki/Gary_Chapman

[55 & 56] https://greatergood.berkeley.edu/article/item/5_ways_giving_is_good_for_you/

Conclusion

[57] http://www.scholarpedia.org/article/Butterfly_effect#Butterfly_effect.2C_causality_and_chance

About the Author

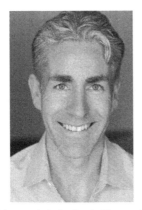

Photography by Jen Stanko Photography

Gregg C. Roberts, INHC, first entered the wellness business working his way through college within the health and fitness industry in southern CA. He has appeared on NBC, CNN, and E! as a guest for various news shows.

He co-founded the Blue Velvet Boxing Club, an award-winning exclusive boxing gym that catered to celebrities and Wall Street executives located in the Flatiron district of NYC. Gregg has been an owner-operator of multiple businesses, from fitness to food, throughout greater NYC ranging from 20-200 employees.

He is the founder and CEO of SimpleWisdom Wellbeing Solutions, LLC, a workplace wellness company focused on improving the overall health and wellbeing of a company's workforce–one employee at a time.

He enjoys serving on a variety of different boards including Stand Together Make A Difference (STMAD), a not-for-profit coalition whose aim is to help prevent substance abuse and addiction through education and awareness. He is also a mentor for at-risk-youth teenagers through Pathways Danbury (CT).

Gregg received his BA from University of California, Santa Barbara, and attended the OPM program at Harvard Business School. He is a graduate of The Institute for Integrative Nutrition in NYC. He is actively involved in the health & wellness sector, enjoys boxing workouts, playing tennis, hiking, and is a father of three children.

To connect with Gregg visit www.GreggCRoberts.com or www.TheSimpleWisdom.com.

Your pathway to wellness is in your hands!
Be a part of our wellbeing community.
Visit *www.GreggCRoberts.com/press* to download
your free PDF and practice my 5 simple lifestyle pillars.

Attain and sustain your optimal health.
Learn how to - P.R.E.S.S. to Success.

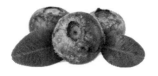

Notes

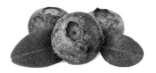

Notes

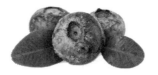

Notes

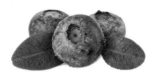

Notes

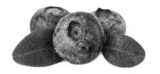

Notes

Made in the USA
Lexington, KY
06 October 2017